Protecting the Kings Table

Daniels guide for being up to ten times healthier, by avoiding harmful food additives, GMO foods and toxic personal care products.

By Daniel W Osborne
Edited by Nancy G Walker, Osborne, Cueto

ISBN-13: 978-0615814278

Made in the USA

To Machelle my patient wife and all of my supportive family and to Whom who gives us mental impressions.

Contents

About this book   V
Legal disclaimer   VII

1. Alphabetical Key to Food Additives................1

2. List of food additives based on European
    numbers or E numbers....................................21

3. Genetically altered foods............................301

4. Possible toxins that may be in personal care
   products...318

5. List of references.......................................327

About this book

This book is a listing of food additives for a reference to check on foods. In addition, there is a compilation of GMO foods to avoid, and a list of toxins found in personal care products.

The list of food additives are in a European number format, which is convenient in terms of grouping them in logical order. There is an alphabetical key to reference the E numbers.

Even trace amounts of food additive toxins may make a person unwell in time and reduce health and strength, especially when older. Use this book to check on food additives and altered foods.

For example, I accidently used toothpaste that had Propylene Glycol (antifreeze) and it made my kidneys ache severely for more than a week before I discovered the cause. For health, it is best to check the ingredients of everything...

VI

The necessary legal disclaimer

In this book, I take on the role of health researcher and information compiler. In this, I am dependent on my resources in being accurate. The information here can be found in other resources including the internet. The value to you is the convenience of having this information readily available. To my knowledge, all information is correct, but it is possible there are mistakes. For any question, I urge further research on your part, especially if you are getting sick for unknown reasons. Seek out professional licensed medical care for any chronic health problem. I suggest finding a Naturopath or an Ecological (Allergy, Environmental, and Nutritional) doctor.

This book has the common adverse reactions to food additives and altered foods. Certain individuals may have uncommon reactions to food additives and altered foods. You may have a bad reaction to something that is not known to give bad reactions.

In the simplest case, a person will ingest item "A", and right after get an obvious bad reaction "B" and know what is going on. However, there are additives that give trace ill effects that may build up in time and these can vary from person to person. You may have a bad reaction to something, which is diffcrent from what is noted in a reference book.

"Thou shalt not eat any abominable thing"   Deuteronomy 14:3

Alphabetical Key to Food Additives. Find the food additive and then use its E-number to look it up on the E-number listing of food additives starting on page 21. Note: E-numbers in bold indicate caution or danger.

Acacia or gum Arabic E414	Acesulphame potassium E950
Acetic acid, glacial E260	Acetic and fatty acid esters of glycerol E472a
Acetone peroxide E929	Acetylated distarch adipate E1422
Acetylated distarch glycerol E1423	Acetylated distarch phosphate E1414
Acetylated oxidised starch E1451	Acid treated starch E1401
Acid Yellow E105	Adipic acid E355
Agar E406	Alginic acid E400
Alitame E956	Alkaline treated starch E1402
Alkanet or Alkannin E103	Allura red AC E129
Aluminium E173	Aluminium, calcium, sodium, magnesium, potassium and ammonium salts of fatty acids E470

Aluminum ammonium sulfate E523	Aluminum potassium sulfate E522
Aluminium silicate E559	Aluminum sodium sulfate E521
Aluminum sulfate E520	Aluminum Stearate E573
Amaranth E123	Ammonium acetate E264
Ammonium adipates E359	Ammonium alginate E403
Ammonium bicarbonate E503	Ammonium chloride E510
Ammonium citrate E380	Ammonium fumarate E368
Ammonium hydrogen carbonate E503	Ammonium hydroxide E527
Ammonium lactate E328	Ammonium malate E349
Ammonium persulfate E923	Ammonium phosphate, dibasic E342
Ammonium phosphate, monobasic or Ammonium dihydrogen phosphates E342	Ammonium polyphosphates E545
Ammonium salts of phosphatidic acid E442	Ammonium stearate E571
Ammonium sulfate E517	α-Amylase E1100
Annatto extracts	Anoxomer

E160b	E323
Anthocyanins or Grape skin extract or Blackcurrant extract E163	Arabinogalactan or larch gum E409
Archil, lacmus E121	Argon E938
Ascorbic acid E300	Ascorbyl palmitate E304
Ascorbyl stearate E305	Aspartame E951
Aspartame-acesulphame salt E962	Azodicarbonamide E927a
Azorubine or Carmoisine E122	b-apo-8' Carotenoic acid methyl or ethyl ester E160f
b-apo-8' Carotenal E160e	Basic methacrylate copolymer E1205
Beeswax, white and yellow E901	Beet red E162
Bentonite E558	Benzoic acid E210
Benzoyl peroxide E928	Benzyl alcohol E1519
Benzylated hydrocarbons E1501	Biphenyl, Diphenyl. E230
Black 7984 E152	Bleached starch E1403
Bone phosphate E542	Borax E285
Brilliant black BN or Brilliant Black PN	Brilliant Blue FCF

E151	E133
Brown FK	Brown HT
E154	E155
Butane	Butane-1,3 diol
E943a	E1502
Butylated hydroxyanisole	Butylated hydroxytoluene
E320	E321
Calcium acetate	Calcium alginate
E263	E404
Calcium aluminium silicate	Calcium ascorbate
E556	E302
Calcium benzoate	Calcium carbonate
E213	E170
Calcium chloride	Calcium citrate
E509	E333
Calcium disodium ethylenediaminetetraacetate or calcium disodium EDTA	Calcium ferrocyanide
E385	E538
Calcium formate	Calcium fumarate
E238	E367
Calcium glycerylphosphate	Calcium gluconate
E383	E578
Calcium glutamate	Calcium guanylate
E623	E629
Calcium hydroxide	Calcium iodate
E526	E916
Calcium inosinate	Calcium lactate
E633	E327

Calcium lactylate E482	Calcium malate E352
Calcium oleyl lactylate E482	Calcium oxide E529
Calcium Hydrogen Sulfite E227	Calcium peroxide E930
Calcium phosphate, dibasic or calcium hydrogen phosphate E341	Calcium phosphate, monobasic or calcium dihydrogen phosphate E341
Calcium phosphate, tribasic E341	Calcium polyphosphates E544
Calcium propionate E282	Calcium 5'-ribonucleotides E634
Calcium silicate

E552 | Calcium sodium polyphosphate E543 |
Calcium sorbate E203	Calcium stearyl fumarate E486
Calcium stearoyl lactylate E482	Calcium sulphate E516
Calcium Sulphite E226	Calcium tartrate E354
Candelilla wax E902	Canthaxanthin E161g
Caramel I E150a	Caramel II E150b
Caramel III E150c	Caramel IV E150d
Carbamide

E927b | Carbon blacks or Vegetable carbon E153 |
| Carbon dioxide | Carnauba wax |

E290	E903
Carotene	Carrageenan
E160a	E407
Cassia gum	Castor Oil
E499	E1503
Cellulose microcrystalline	Cellulose, powdered
E460	E460
Chloropentafluoroethane	Chlorophyll
E945	E140
Chlorophyll-copper complex	Chlorophyllin copper complex, sodium and potassium salts E141
E141	
Chlorine	Chlorine dioxide
E925	E926
Cholic acid	Choline salts
E1000	E1001
C.I. 13015 or C.I. 14270	Citric acid
E105	E330
Citric and fatty acid esters of glycerol	Cochineal or carmines or carminic acid
E472c	E120
Cupric sulphate	Curcumin or turmeric
E519	E100
Cyclamate or calcium cyclamate or sodium cyclamate	Danish agar
E952	E408
Dehydroacetic acid	Dextrin roasted starch
E265	E1400
Diacetyltartaric and fatty acid esters of glycerol	Dicalcium diphosphate
E472e	E540

Dichlorodifluoromethane, or (common brand name) Freon-12 E940	Dimethyl dicarbonate E242
Dioctyl sodium sulphosuccinate E480	Dipotassium guanylate E628
Dipotassium inosinate E632	Disodium 5'-ribonucleotides E635
Disodium 5'-guanylate E627	Disodium 5'-inosinate E631
Distarch phosphate E1412	Dodecyl gallate E312
Distarch glycerine E1430	Distarch glycerol E1411
Enzyme treated starches E1405	Erythorbic acid E315
Erythorbin acid E317	Erythritol E968
Erythrosine E127	Esters of Colophane E915
Esterified soy oil E479b	Ethanol E1510
Ethoxylated Mono- and Di- Glycerides E488	Ethoxyquin E324
Ethyl Acetate E1504	Ethyl gallate E313
Ethyl lauroyl arginate E243	Ethyl maltol E637
Ethylparaben	(Ethyl para-hydroxybenzoate)

E214	E214
Extracts of Rosemary E392	Fast green FCF E143
Fast Yellow AB E105	Fast Yellow E105
Ferric ammonium citrate E381	Ferrous carbonate E505
Ferrous hexacyanomanganate E537	Ferrous gluconate E579
Ferrous lactate E585	Flavin mononucleotide (FMN) E106
Flavoxanthin E161a	Food Yellow 2 E105
Formaldehyde E240	Formic acid E236
Fumaric acid E297	Furcellaran E408
Gellan gum E418	Gluconic acid E574
Glucono δ-lactone or Glucono delta-lactone E575	Glucose oxidase E1102
L-glutamic acid E620	Glycerin or glycerol E422
Glycerol esters of wood rosins E445	Glycerol diacetate E1517
Glycerol monoacetate E1516	Glycerol monoacetin E1516
Glycine E640	Glycyrrhizin E958
Gold	Green S

E175	E142
Guaiac Gum	Guanylic acid
E314	E626
Guar gum	Gum benzoic
E412	E906
4-hexylresorcinol	Heptylparaben (Heptyl para-hydroxybenzoate)
E586	E209
Helium	Heptonolactone 1, 4
E939	E370
Hexamine	Hydrochloric acid
E239	E507
Hydrogen	Hydroxy ethyl cellulose
E949	E1524
Hydroxypropyl cellulose	Hydroxy propyl distarch glycerine E1441
E463	
Hydroxypropyl distarch phosphate	Hydroxypropyl methylcellulose
E1442	E464
Hydroxypropyl starch	Indanthrene blue RS
E1440	E130
Indigotine	Inosinic acid
E132	E630
Invertase	Iron oxide
E1103	E172
Isobutane	Isomalt
E943b	E953
Isopropyl citrate	Karaya gum
E384	E416
Kryptoxanthin	Lanolin
E161c	E913
L-cysteine	L-cysteine hydrochloride monohydrate

E910	E921
L-cysteine monohydrochloride E920	L-Leucine E641
Lactic acid E270	Lactic and fatty acid esters of glycerol E472b
Lactitol E966	Lactylated fatty acid esters of glycerol and propane E478
Lecithin E322	Lecithin citrate E344
Lipases 1104	Locust bean gum or carob bean gum E410
Lutein E161b	Lycopene E160d
Lysine E642	Lysine hydrochloride E642
Lysozyme E1105	Magnesium carbonate E504
Magnesium chloride E511	Magnesium gluconate E580
Magnesium citrate E345	Magnesium glutamate E625
Magnesium hydroxide E528	Magnesium lactate E329
Magnesium oxide E530	Magnesium phosphate, dibasic E343
Magnesium phosphate, monobasic E343	Magnesium phosphate, tribasic 343
Magnesium	Magnesium silicate or

pyrophosphate E546	Talc E553
Magnesium stearate E572	Magnesium sulphate E518
Malic acid E296	Maltitol and maltitol syrup or hydrogenated glucose syrup E965
Maltol E636	Mannitol E421
Metatartaric acid E353	Methyl esters of fatty acids E911
Methyl ethyl cellulose E465	Methyl cellulose E461
Methyl glucoside E489	Methylparaben or Methyl-p-hydroxy-benzoate E218
Microcystalline wax 905 E	Mineral oil E905a
Mixed tartaric, acetic and fatty acid esters of glycerol' or 'tartaric, acetic and fatty acid esters of glycerol (mixed) E472f	Mono- and di-glycerides of fatty acids E471
Monoammonium L-glutamate E624	Monopotassium L-glutamate E622
Monosodium L-glutamate or MSG E621	Monostarch phosphate E1410
Montanic acid esters (fat with alcohol)	Natamycin or pimaricin E235

E912	
Neohesperidine dihydrochalcone E959	Neotame E961
Niacin E375	Nisin E234
Nitrogen E931	Nitrogen E941
Nitrogen oxides E918	Nitrogen trichloride E919
Nitrous oxide E932	Nitrous oxide E942
Octafluorocyclobutane E946	Octyl gallate E311
Orthophenyl phenol, E231	2-Phenylphenol E231
Orcein, Orchil E121	Oxidised polyethylene E914
Oxidised starch E1404	Oxygen E948
Oxystearin E387	Paprika oleoresins E160c
Paraffins E905	Partial polyglycerol esters of polycondensed fatty acids of castor oil E498
Patent blue V E131	Pectin E440
Perlite E599	Petrolatum or petroleum jelly E905b
Phosphated distarch phosphate E1413	Phosphoric acid E338

Polydextrose E1200	Polydimethylsiloxane or Dimethylpolysiloxane E900a
Polyethylene glycol 8000 E1521	Polyglycerol esters of fatty acids E45
Polyglycerol esters of interesterified ricinoleic acid E476	Polyoxyethylene (40) stearate E431
Polysorbate 60 or Polyoxyethylene (20) sorbitan monostearate E435	Polysorbate 65 or Polyoxyethylene (20) sorbitan tristearate E436
Polysorbate 80 or Polyoxyethylene (20) sorbitan monooleate E433	Polyvinylpyrrolidone E1201
Polyvinylpolypyrrolidone E1202	Polyoxypropylene-polyoxyethylene polymers E497
Ponceau 4R E124	Potassium acetate or potassium diacetate E261
Potassium adipate E357	Potassium alginate E402
Potassium aluminium silicate E555	Potassium ascorbate E303
Potassium benzoate E212	Potassium bicarbonate E501
Potassium bisulphite	Potassium bromate

E228	E924
Potassium carbonate E501	Potassium chloride E508
Potassium citrate E332	Potassium dihydrogen citrate E332
Potassium ferrocyanide E536	Potassium fumarate E366
Potassium gluconate E577	Potassium hydroxide E525
Potassium iodate E917	Potassium lactate E326
Potassium malate E351	Potassium metabisulphite E224
Potassium nitrate E252	Potassium nitrite E249
Potassium persulfate E922	Potassium phosphate, dibasic E340
Ponceau SX E125	Ponceau 6R E126
Potassium phosphate, monobasic E340	Potassium phosphate, tribasic E340
Potassium polymetaphosphate E452	Potassium propionate E283
Potassium pyrophosphate E450	Potassium silicate E560
Potassium sodium tartrate E337	Potassium sorbate E202

Potassium sulphate E515	Potassium sulphite E225
Potassium tartrate or Potassium acid tartrate E336	Potassium tripolyphosphate E451
Processed eucheuma seaweed E407a	Propane E944
Propane- 1,2-diol or Propylene glycol E490	
Propionic acid E280	Propyl gallate E310
Propylene glycol E1520	Propylene glycol alginate E405
Propylene glycol mono - and di-esters or Propylene glycol esters of fatty acidsm E477	Propylparaben or Propyl-p-hydroxy-benzoate E216
Proteases (papain, bromelain, ficin) E1101	Pullulan E1204
Quillaia extract E999	Quinoline yellow E104
Citrus Red 2 E121	Red 2G E128
Refined microcrystalline wax E907	Rhodoxanthin E161f
Riboflavin E101	Riboflavin 5'-phosphate sodium E101
Rice bran wax E908	Rubixanthin E161d

Saccharin or calcium saccharine or sodium saccharine or potassium saccharine E954	Saffron or crocetin or crocin E164
Shellac E904	Silicon dioxide, amorphous E551
Silver E174	Sodium acetate E262
Sodium alginate E401	Sodium aluminium phosphate E541
Sodium aluminosilicate E554	Sodium ascorbate E301
Sodium benzoate E211	Sodium bicarbonate E500
Sodium Biphenyl-2-yl Oxide E232	Sodium bisulphite E222
Sodium carbonate E500	Sodium carboxymethylcellulose E466
Sodium citrate E331	Sodium Dehydroacetate E266
Sodium diacetate E262	Sodium dihydrogen citrate or Monosodium citrate E331
Sodium ethyl para-Hydroxybenzoate E215	
Sodium erythorbate E 316/318	Sodium ferrocyanide E535
Sodium formate	Sodium fumarate

E237	E365
Sodium gluconate	Sodium hydroxide
E576	E524
Sodium hydrogen malate	Sodium lactate
E350	E325
Sodium lactylate	Sodium lauryl sulfate
E481	E487
Sodium malate	Sodium metabisulphite
E350	E223
Sodium metaphosphate, insoluble	Sodium methyl para-hydroxybenzoate
E452	E219
Sodium nitrate	Sodium nitrite
E251	E250
Sodium oleyl lactylate	Sodium phosphate, dibasic E339
E481	
Sodium phosphate, monobasic E339	Sodium phosphate, tribasic E339
Sodium polyphosphates, glassy E452	Sodium propionate
	E281
Sodium propyl para-hydroxybenzoate	Sodium pyrophosphate
E217	E450
Sodium silicate	Sodium sorbate
E550	E201
Sodium stearyl fumarate	Sodium stearoyl lactylate
E485	E481
Sodium sulphate	Sodium sulphite
E514	E221
Sodium tartrate	Sodium thiosulfate
E335	E539
Sodium tripolyphosphate	Sorbic acid

E451	E200
Sorbitan monolaurate E493	Sorbitan monooleate E494
Sorbitan monopalmitate E495	Sorbitan monostearate E491
Sorbitan trioleat E496	Sorbitan tristearate E492
Sorbitol or sorbitol syrup E420	Spermaceti wax E909
Spiramycin E710	Stannous chloride E512
Starch acetate E1420	Starch Acetate Esterified with Vinyl Acetate E1421
Starch sodium octenylsuccinate E1450 E1450	Stearic acid or fatty acid E570
Stearyl citrate E484	Stearyl Tartrate E483
Steviol glycosides E960	Succinic acid E363
Sucralose E955	Sucroglycerides E474
Sucrose acetate isobutyrate E444	Sucrose esters of fatty acids E473
Sulfuric acid E513	Sulphur dioxide E220
Sunset yellow FCF E110	Synthetic calcium aluminates E598
Tannic acid or tannins E181	Tara gum E417
Tartaric acid	Tartaric acid esters of monoglycerides and

	diglycerides of fatty acids.
E334	E472d
Tartrazine E102	tert-Butylhydroquinone E319
Thaumatin E957	Thiabendazole E233
Thiodipropionic acid E388	Titanium dioxide E171
α-Tocopherol E307	δ-Tocopherol E309
γ-Tocopherol E308	Tocopherols concentrate, mixed E306
Tragacanth gum E413	Triacetin E1518
Triammonium citrate E380	Triethyl citrate E1505
Tylosin E713	Violoxanthin E161e
Xanthan gum E415	Xanthophyll E161
Xylitol E967	Yellow 5 E102
Zinc acetate E650	Zinc silicate E557

Coloring E100-E181:

A food coloring is an additive when put into food will change or make its color better. Colorings can be natural or synthetically created from plants, herbs or even insects. Generally, colorings are not acutely harmful to most people, but some people have noticeable reactions.

Natural colors are not required to be tested by a number of regulatory bodies throughout the world; however these may have substances with synthetic origins. In addition just because something is considered natural does not mean it can't create harmful reactions for some people.

Norway had a general ban on all food colorings since 1978 due to adverse reactions especially with children. However Norway rescinded that ban due to new trade rules with the European Union in 2001; but implemented labeling all food colors so consumers in Norway can make their own choices. EU rules do not require such product labeling.

Note: The E-Numbers in bold indicate caution or danger.

E100	$C_{21}H_{20}O_6$
Curcumin.	It is the purified compound from the root and stem of the Yellowroot, which is a plant of the ginger family
(Curcumin is the principle spice in	which grows in tropical South Asia. Annually Yellowroot is picked, boiled, and crushed into a

Turmeric.) Color - Yellow and Orange.	yellow/orange powder. Turmeric has been used historically as a component of Indian Ayurvedi medicine since 1900 BC to treat a wide variety of ailments. Curcumin is responsible for most of the biological activity of turmeric. Curcumin is used in curry powders, cheeses, salad dressings, yogurt, orange juice, biscuits, sauces, baked products, canned beverages, pickles, butter, margarine, and relishes. It is still being evaluated regarding reproductive toxicity. As with any powerful spice or herb be cautious of excessive daily usage, seems safe enough in proper gentle use. It has many helpful effects but watch for side effects. For instance curcuma is known to inhibit blood clotting; it should be avoided for a two week period before major surgery and not used in conjunction with blood thinners. It is known to aggravate gallstone problems. It is a possible risk to conception and may cause cancer. Listed for UK, NZ, AU, and EU. Not listed in USA and CAN, but Turmeric is listed.
E101 **Riboflavin, commonly**	$C_{17}H_{20}N_4O_6$ Vitamin, all listed information indicates it is safe. It makes up most of the color in B vitamins, and the

known as (Vitamin B2). Color - Yellow and Orange.	yellow color in urine from B vitamins. Exposure to light destroys riboflavin. A good additive to prevent a common deficiency. Signs of severe B2 deficiency include cracked and red lips, inflammation of the lining of mouth and tongue, mouth ulcers, cracks at the corners of the mouth and sore throat. A deficiency in B2 usually a general overall deficiency. Used in breakfast cereals, pastas, baby foods, fruit drinks processed cheese and vitamin-enriched milk products. Listed for CAN, NZ, UK, AU, EU and USA.
E102 **Tartrazine or FD&C Yellow No:5 or Yellow 5 or CI Acid Yellow23 or CI Food Yellow 4. or Coal tar dye or Polycyclic**	$C_{16}H_9N_4Na_3O_9S_2$ It is synthetically produced. May increase hyperactivity in children, and asthmatics can react badly. It may cause or aggravate hay fever, skin rashes, blurred vision. Known to provoke asthma attacks; can cause altered states of perception and altered behavior, such as uncontrolled hyper agitation and confusion; wakefulness in young children, may cause cancer. It is known to inhibit zinc metabolism and interfere with digestive enzymes. An estimation (in Wikipedia) is about .12% of USA population will have some kind of reaction. About .01% will have hives. Used in colored fizzy

Aromatic Hydrocarbon. Color - Yellow and Orange.	drinks, soups, cake mixes, ice-cream, custard power, chewing gum, fruit, honey products, yogurt, noodles, pickles, flavored chips and many convenient fast foods. Avoid, especially if sensitive to aspirin. Previously banned in Norway and others. Listed for CAN, NZ, AU, EU, UK, JPN and USA. *These additives should be avoided by children especially if have attention problems. (E110), quinoline yellow (E104), carmoisine (E122), allura red (E129), tartrazine (E102) and ponceau 4R (E124)*
E103 **Alkanet or Alkannin or (Chrysoine resorcinol)** Color - Yellow and Orange.	$C_{16}H_{16}O_5$ Alkanet is a natural red color derived from the root of Alkanna tinctoria plant, which grows in southern France and on the shores of Levant France. Used to color wines and foods, and imparts a port-wine color. Asthmatics can react badly, and may increase hyperactivity in children. Avoid, especially if sensitive to aspirin. Listed for AU, CAN and USA. Not listed for EU and UK.
E104 **Quinoline Yellow or D&C Yellow**	$C_{18}H_{13}NO_{5/8/11}S_{1/2}$ Made from the disodium salt of disulphonic acid. It may increase hyperactivity in children, also may decrease intelligence of children. May cause the intake of extra

No:10. **or** **Food Yellow** **13** **or** **C.I. 47005** **or** **Quinoline** **Yellow WS.** Color - Yellow and Orange.	aluminum. May cause genetic mutation, inflammation of skin, skin rash, asthma, and stuffy nose. Used in cough drops, smoked fish, lipsticks, hair products, colognes. In a wide range of medications. Not listed for CAN and USA. Listed for AU, NZ, EU and UK. *(These should be avoided by children especially those with attention problems. (E110), quinoline yellow (E104), carmoisine (E122), allura red (E129), tartrazine (E102) and ponceau 4R (E124))*
E105 **Fast Yellow** **AB or Fast** **Yellow, Acid** **Yellow or** **C.I. 13015 or** **C.I. 14270** **or Food** **Yellow 2.** Yellow color.	$C_{12}H_{11}N_3O_6S_2$ An azo dye. It is used as a food dye. It is now not listed for CAN, UK, EU, NZ, AU and USA, not used anymore, because toxicological data shows it is harmful.
E106 **Riboflavin -** **5'-sodium** **phosphate** **or** **Flavin**	$C_{17}H_{21}N_4O_9P$ The molecule consists mainly of the monosodium salt of the 5'-monophosphate ester of riboflavin dihydrate obtained from chemical action on E101 riboflavin. It is rapidly turned to free riboflavin after

mononucleo tide (FMN). Yellow-orange color. Vitamin supplement, Food fortifier.	ingestion. It is found in many foods for babies and young children. Used in breakfast cereals, pastas, baby foods, fruit drinks processed cheese, jam, sugar products, and vitamin-enriched milk products. No reported bad effects listed in sources, considering the need to keep inside safe guidelines. Not listed for UK, CAN, NZ, AU and EU. Listed for USA.
E107 **Yellow 2G.** Yellow color.	$C_{16}H_{10}Na_2N_4O_7S_2$ A synthetic yellow azo dye, made from coal tar. Used in mayonnaise, drinks, and soft drinks, soluble in water. It may cause asthma, rashes and hyperactivity. People sensitive to aspirin and asthma sufferers should avoid it. Limit usage if possible. Not listed for CAN, EU, UK, AU, NZ and USA and many others.
E110 **FD&C Yellow No:6** **or** **Sunset Yellow FCF** **or**	$C_{16}H_{10}N_2Na_2O_7S_2$ Manufactured from aromatic hydrocarbons from petroleum. A synthetic coal tar and an azo yellow dye which is useful in fermented foods which must be heat treated. It may be found in orange sodas, Swiss rolls, apricot jam, citrus marmalade, sweets, beverage mix and packet soups, margarine, custard powders, packaged lemon gelatin desserts, energy drinks, medications including

Orange Yellow S **or** **CI Food yellow 3** Color - Yellow and Orange.	over the counter medications. May increase hyperactivity in affected children. Take care if you are sensitive to aspirin. On September 9, 2011 the European Union announced that they would consider reducing the maximum permitted concentration of sunset yellow (in drinks) from 50mg/L to 20mg/L. The proposed change to be adopted by the end of the year. http://www.bbc.co.uk/news/uk-scotland-scotland-business-14857275 . Previously banned in Norway. Listed for UK, CAN, EU, NZ, AU, UK, JPN and USA. *These should be avoided by children especially those with attention problems. (E110), quinoline yellow (E104), carmoisine (E122), allura red (E129), tartrazine (E102) and ponceau 4R (E124)*
E111 **Orange GGN.** Orange color.	$C_{16}H_{10}N_2Na_2O_7S_2$ It is the disodium salt of 1-(m-sulfophenylazo)-2-naphthol-6-sulfonic acid. It is currently not listed for UK, AU, NZ, EU, USA, CAN and most other countries because research data shows it is harmful.
E120 **Cochineal**	$C_{22}H_{20}O_{13}$ A natural red color, made from the insect Dayctylopius coccus, which

or Carminic acid or Carmines. Color - Red	feeds off various cacti plants. A natural red color is obtained by crushing of the female Dactilopius coccus, a cactus-dwelling insect indigenous to Central America. The dye is expensive due to the quantity of shells required to produce a small amount. Used in alcoholic beverages, dyed cheeses, puddings, icings, sweets, sauces, fizzy drinks, cakes, soups and pie fillings. May increase hyperactivity in children. May be toxic to embryos. May cause other bad reactions. Listed for CAN, AU, NZ, UK, EU and USA.
E121 **Orcein or Orchil.** Orange to yellow color also can be a dark red powder	$C_{28}H_{24}N_2O_7$. Several synthetic food dyes are made from a species of lichen commonly known as "orchella weeds". Citrus Red 2 also made from this family of lichen is used in the USA to coat oranges, this dye is considered cancer causing, but should not penetrate through the orange peel to the pulp. Orcein is a reddish-brown dye, orchil is a purple-blue dye. Other non food uses are microscope slides and in clothes. Listed for CAN, USA. Not listed for NZ, UK, EU, and AU. *These should be avoided by children especially those with attention problems. (E110), quinoline yellow (E104), carmoisine*

E122	(E122), allura red (E129), tartrazine (E102) and ponceau 4R (E124)
E122 **Carmoisine, Azorubine** **or** **Food Red 3** **Azorubin S** **or** **Brillantcar moisin O** **or** **Acid Red 14** **or** **C.I. 14720.** Color – Red.	$C_{20}H_{12}N_2Na_2O_7S_2$ A synthetic azo dye made from coal tar. Used in jams, jellies, preserves, breadcrumbs, puddings, cakes, sweets, brown sauce, and cheesecake mixes. It may be carcinogenic, may cause or increase hyperactivity in children, may cause a skin rash similar to a rash from nettles, may cause skin swelling. Asthmatics can react badly. Especially avoid if sensitive to aspirin. Not listed in USA, JPN, and CAN. Listed for NZ, AU, UK and EU.
E123 **Amaranth** **or** **Red No. 2** **or** **FD&C Red No. 2,** **or** **E123, C.I. Food Red 9** **or** **Acid Red 27** **or** **Azorubin S,** **or**	$C_{20}H_{11}N_2Na_3O_{10}S_3$ Amaranth is a cosmopolitan genus of herbs. Approximately 60 species are recognized, with inflorescences and foliage color ranging from purple and red to gold. Several species are grown as a grain for food. The flowers of the 'Hopi Red Dye' amaranth are the source of the red dye, it is also made synthetically from coal tar. Used in soups, truffles, jelly, jams, gravy granules, ice-creams, and canned fruit pie fillings. A suspected carcinogen and mutagen, May increase hyperactivity in children.

C.I. 16185. Color – Red.	Avoid if sensitive to aspirin. Not listed in Russia and Ukraine. Listed for CAN, UK, AU, NZ, EU, JPN and USA.
E124 **Ponceau 4R** **or** **Cochineal** **Red A** **or** **Brilliant** **Scarlet 4R.** Color – Red.	$C_{20}H_{11}N_2Na_3O_{10}S_3$ A synthetic azo dye made from coal tar. Used in truffles, jellies, canned strawberries and fruit pie fillings, salami, cake mixes, soups, and dessert toppings. Causes cancer in animals, can produce bad reactions in asthmatics and people allergic to aspirin; 1 in 10,000 people are allergic. Linked to hyperactivity in children. Not listed in CAN, and USA. Listed for EU, AU, NZ, UK and JPN. *These should be avoided by children especially those with attention problems. (E110), quinoline yellow (E104), carmoisine (E122), allura red (E129), tartrazine (E102) and ponceau 4R*
E125 **Ponceau SX** **or** **Scarlet GN** **or** **C.I. Food** **Red 1 or** **FD&C Red** **No. 4 or** **C.I. 14700.**	$Na_2C_{18}H_{14}N_2S_2O_7$ It usually comes as a disodium salt. It is permitted in fruit peels and maraschino cherries. Caution, not much information. It is indicated that half of a rodent population will be killed by a dosage greater than 5 gm per Kg. (a very large dose). http://www.drugfuture.com/toxic/q42-q313.html Not listed for UK, EU, NZ, AU and

	USA. Listed for CAN
Color-Red.	
E126 **Ponceau 6R, or Crystal ponceau 6R or Crystal scarlet or Brilliant crystal scarlet 6R or Acid Red 44, or C.I. 16250.** Color – Red.	$C_{20}H_{12}N_2Na_2O_7S_2$ A synthetic azo dye which yields a red color and usually comes as a disodium salt. Soluble in water. Can be used in maraschino cherries and on fruit peels in some countries. Not much information on safety. Not listed for UK, NZ, AU, USA, EU and CAN.
E127 **Erythrosine BS** **or** **Red No. 3.** Color – Red.	$C_{20}H_6I_4Na_2O_5$ Coal tar dye, organoiodine compound, specifically a derivative of fluorine It is a cherry-pink synthetic primarily used for food coloring. Used in cake frosting, cake-decorating gels, canned fruit, cherries, custard mix, pate, stuffed olives, biscuits, and chocolate. It is a disodium salt. May cause sensitivity to light and learning difficulties; can increase thyroid hormone levels and lead to hyperthyroidism, was shown to cause thyroid cancer in rats in a 1990 study. May increase hyperactivity in children. Listed for

	JPN, CAN, EU, UK, AU, NZ and USA.
E128 **Red 2G.** Color - Red.	$C_{18}H_{13}N_3Na_2O_8S_2$ A synthetic red coal tar and azo dye. Used only in breakfast sausages with a minimum cereal content of 6% and burger meat with a minimum vegetable and/or cereal content of 4%. (The bright red hamburger meat you feel good about buying in the store may have this dye or some other dye, natural meat is usually grey in color) To be avoided by hyperactive people, asthmatics and aspirin sensitive people. Also a risk of skin rash and anemia. Possibly carcinogenic when added to foods. In the intestines, Red 2G can be converted to the toxic compound aniline, so there are concerns Red 2G may ultimately interfere with blood hemoglobin, as well as cause cancer. Not listed for USA, JPN, Switzerland, CAN, NZ, EU, AU and UK.
E129 **Allura red AC or Allura Red or Food Red 17 or C.I. 16035**	$C_{18}H_{14}N_2Na_2O_8S_2$ Originally manufactured from coal tar, but is now mostly made from petroleum. Introduced in the early eighties to replace amaranth (E123) which is considered not safe. Used in condiments, medications, sweets, and drinks. It is thought that any allergic reaction to this dye is small

or FD&C Red 40. Color - Red, Orange	as compared to reactions to other azo dyes. Connected to cancer in mice, linked to thyroid abnormality, brain dysfunction, hyperactivity in children and light sensitivity. Listed for CAN, JPN, UK, AU, EU and USA. Once was not listed (or banned) in many nations.
E130 **Indanthrene blue RS.** Color-Blue.	$C_{28}H_{14}N_2O_4$ Indanthrene blue RS is a synthetic anthraquinone dye. It is used to dye cotton and as a pigment in high quality paints and enamels. No known common food usage, not much information. Not listed for UK, CAN, EU, AU, NZ and USA.
E131 **Patent Blue V or Food Blue 5 or Sulphan Blue.** Color – Blue	$C27H31N2NaO6S2$ A synthetic blue-violet coal tar dye seldom used in the food industry. It is a sodium or calcium salt and has the appearance of a violet powder. It is mainly used medically as an blood dye to color the lymph vessels, and the cardiovascular system. Hypersensitivity reactions reported include itching and nettle rash, nausea, low blood pressure, and in rare cases anaphylactic shock. In food it can be used in scotch eggs (a hard boiled egg covered with meat, served cold). Not listed for AU, JPN, NZ, CAN and USA. Listed for EU and UK.

E132 **Indigo Carmine or Idigotine or FD&C Blue #2.** Color – Blue.	$C_{16}H_8N_2Na_2O_8S_2$ Synthetic coal tar dye. It is used as a pH indicator, blue at pH 11.4 and yellow at pH 13.0. Commonly added to tablets and capsules. It is also used in ice cream, sweets, baked goods, confectionary, biscuits. A suspected carcinogen, may cause hyperactivity, nausea, breathing difficulty, skin reactions, increased blood pressure. Listed for JPN, NZ, CAN, EU, AU, UK and USA.
E133 **Brilliant Blue FCF or FD&C Blue Dye No:1 or CI Acid blue 9 or CI Food blue 2 or CI Pigment blue 24.** Color-Blue	$C_{37}H_{34}N_2Na_2O_9S_3$ It can be combined with tartrazine (E102) to produce various shades of green. It is used in dairy products, sweets, processed peas, ice-cream, and drinks, also in hygiene, and cosmetics applications. Suspected carcinogen, linked to hyperactivity, asthmatics should avoid as it may trigger a reaction. Can be inside almost any processed product even in concentrations less than one percent, which may not be on product label. Caution. Listed for CAN,USA, JPN, EU, UK, NZ and AU.
E140 **Chlorophyll** Color – Green.	$C_{55}H_{70}O_6N_4Mg$ Green color occurs naturally in all plants. Chlorophyll is used as a source of olive/dark-green color, it is susceptible to fading. Chlorophyll powder is not soluble in water, and it

	is first mixed with a small quantity of vegetable oil to obtain the desired solution. Used in soaps, preserved fruits, vegetables, sweets, soups, ice cream, sauce mixes and medicines. Chlorophyll is a healthy natural "green" substance for nutrition and cleansing. No known bad effects listed in sources. Listed for CAN, EU, AU, NZ, UK and USA.
E141 **Copper complexes of** **1.chlorophyll** **2.Chlorophyllins (Copper Phaephytins).** Color – Green.	$C_{55}H_{70}O_6N_4Cu$ Olive color made or extracted from alfalfa, grass, and nettles. The Mg ion in chlorophyll is substituted by Cu to give a more stable olive green coloring. This makes (1) an "olive green" oil soluble color, or (2) a water soluble green color. Used in cheese, parsley sauce, ice-cream, soups, chewing gum, green vegetables and fruits preserved in liquids. No known bad effects listed in sources. Listed for UK, AU, NZ and EU. Not listed for USA and CAN.
E142 **Green S / Acid Brilliant Green BS.**	$C_{27}H_{25}N_2NaO_7S_2$ Synthetic coal tar dye. Used in canned peas, mint jelly, sauces, packet bread crumbs and cake mixes. It may cause cancer, hypersensitivity, allergic reactions, asthmatics should avoid. Children should avoid,

Color – Green.	especially if hyperactive. Listed for AU, NZ, UK, EU. Not listed for USA, JPN and CAN.
E143 **Fast Green FCF or Food green 3 or FD&C Green No. 3 or Green 1724 or Solid Green FCF or C.I. 42053**. Color- Sea Green.	$C_{37}H_{37}N_2O_{10}S_3+$ A triarylmethane food dye. Its use as a food dye is prohibited in the European Union and some other countries. It can be used for tinned green peas and other vegetables, jellies, sauces, fish, desserts, and dry bakery mixes up to 100 mg/kg. In the United States, Fast Green FCF is the least used of the seven main FDA approved dyes. This substance has been found to have tumor generating effects in experimental animals, as well as mutation causing effects in both experimental animals and humans. http://fscimage.fishersci.com/msds/60270.htm Listed for CAN, JPN, UK, AU, NZ, EU, and USA. Not listed for UK.
E150 **Caramel (a, b, c, d).** Color - Brown and Black.	Emulsifier in soft drinks. Caramel (a,b,c,d) is made by carefully controlled heat treatment of carbohydrates (sugars), in the presence of acids, alkalis, or salts, in a process called caramelization. Color ranges from pale yellow to amber to dark brown. Used in puddings, barley sugar, praline, custard, colas, vinegar, doughnuts,

	crisps, sauces, chocolate, brandy, bread, beer, pancakes and many others. 150b to 150c are linked to gastro-intestinal problems and hypersensitivity. 150a seems fairly safe because it is made without chemicals when heated. You may want to avoid E150b to E150d. Testing continues with E150a. Also caramel coloring may be derived from a variety of source products that are themselves common allergens, such as lactose (from milk), dextrose (usually derived from corn), starch hydrolysates (from corn or wheat), and malt syrup (usually derived from barley). Listed for CAN, AU, NZ, EU, UK and USA.
E151 **Brilliant Black BN or Brilliant Black PN or Brilliant Black A or Black PN or Food Black 1 or Naphthol Black or C.I. Food Brown 1 or**	$C_{28}H_{17}N_5Na_4O_{14}S_4$ A synthetic coal tar and azo dye. Used in food decorations and coatings, desserts, sweets, ice cream, mustard, red fruit jams, soft drinks, flavored milk drinks, fish paste, lumpfish caviar and other foods. May increase hyperactivity in children, may cause hives, and a increase of symptoms for those with sinus problems or stuffy nose. Linked to bowel disorders. People with an aspirin allergy should avoid, as well as asthmatics. Listed for UK, AU, NZ and EU. Not listed for USA, CAN and

C.I. 28440. Color - Brown and Black.	JPN.
E152 **Black 7984 or Food Black 2 or C.I. 27755.** Color – Brown to Black.	$C_{26}H_{19}N_5Na_4O_{13}S_4$ A brown-to-black synthetic diazo dye. It is often used as the tetrasodium salt. It may cause allergic or intolerance reactions, particularly amongst those with an aspirin intolerance. May worsen the symptoms of asthma and hyperactivity in children. Children should avoid. Not listed for CAN, AU, NZ, USA, UK and EU.
E153 **Carbon Black or Vegetable Carbon or (Charcoal).** Color - Brown and Black.	C A natural black color from burnt plant material or incomplete combustion of heavy petroleum products such as FCC tar, coal tar, ethylene cracking tar, and a small amount from vegetable oil. It is used in jam, jelly crystal and liquorices. It may increase hyperactivity in affected children, and cause cancer. Be cautious if you suffer from allergies or intolerances. Note: Pure carbon or charcoal made correctly from burnt plant material is safe and be used medicinally. Listed for AU, NZ, CAN, UK and EU. Not listed for USA.

E154 **Brown FK or Kipper Brown or Chocolate Brown FK or C.I. Food Brown 1.** Color – Brown to Black.	$C_{27}H_{18}N_4Na_2O_9S_2$ A combination of six different synthetic azo dyes with sodium chloride and/or sodium sulfate. It is mainly used to give fish flesh a healthy pigment which will not leach or fade during cooking. Typical products include smoked and cured fish, crisps, hams and cooked meats. It can provoke allergic reactions in people sensitive to salicylates, and may intensify the symptoms of asthma. Children should avoid, same when combined with common meat preservatives benzoates (E210-E213). Listed for EU and UK. Not listed for CAN, NZ, AU and USA.
E155 **Brown HT or Chocolate Brown HT or Food Brown 3 C.I. 20285.** Color - Brown.	$C_{27}H_{18}N_4Na_2O_9S_2$ A coal tar and azo dye. Used in milk, chocolate cakes, chocolate drinks, jams, fish, yoghurts and cheeses. Can produce bad reactions in asthmatics and people allergic to aspirin, known to induce skin sensitivity. It is cancer causing, and has mutating effects. Attention deficit (ADD) children should avoid. Listed for NZ, EU, UK, AU. Not listed for USA, CAN and JPN.
E160a **Carotene, -**	$C_{40}H_{56}$ Naturally inside carrots, tomatoes, apricots, oranges, and greens. It can

Alpha, Beta, Gamma. Color – Orange to Yellow, a Carotene derivative. Supplement.	be extracted from natural sources, but usually made synthetically. The human body converts it to Vitamin A in the liver. Used in fruit juices and squashes, cakes, desserts, butter and margarine etc. No known bad effects in listed sources. Considered safe with proper usage. Listed for UK, CAN, AU, NZ, EU, and USA.
E160b **Annatto or Bixin or Norbixin.** Color – Red, Peach, Yellow.	Carotene derivative, a natural color which is extracted from the seeds of the Annatto tree and yields a dye, red, peach, or yellow in color. Annatto is the crude extract, bixin is the fat-soluble color, and norbixin is the water-soluble color. They are used in lipstick, cosmetics, butter, margarine, soft drinks, pastry, smoked fish, cakes, flavored instant mashed potato, meat balls, mayonnaise, sponge cakes, pudding custards, and yogurt etc. Can cause or aggravate health problems such as hives (skin rash), skin swelling, asthma, hyperactivity, behavior and learning problems in children. Can be labeled as a "natural" ingredient. Commonly used in many products, consider limiting or avoiding, especially if sensitive. Listed for CAN, UK, EU, AU, NZ and USA.
E160c	$C_{40}H_{56}O_3$ (Capsanthin),

Paprika extract or Capsanthin or Capsorubin. Color −Red, Carotene derivative.	$C_{40}H_{56}O_4$ (Capsorubin). Paprika extract is made from the seeds and pods of the red pepper Capsicum annuum. It is a red to orange "spice", extraction is performed by percolation of the seeds and pods in a variety of solvents, primarily hexane, which is removed prior to use. They are used in cheese, orange juice, spice mixtures, sauces, sweets and emulsified processed meats. In poultry feed, it is used to deepen the color of egg yolks. Linked to gastro-intestinal problems, and hypersensitivity, caution. Listed for CAN, EU, NZ, UK, and AU. Not listed for USA.
E160d **Lycopene.** Color − Yellow, Red. Darotene derivative.	$C_{40}H_{56}$ Derived from natural sources, commercially it is isolated from tomatoes and this makes a dark red food color. Used in Spanish foods, Serrano ham and sauces etc. No known bad effects listed in sources. Listed for EU, AU, NZ, UK and USA. Not listed for CAN.
E160e **Beta-apo-8-carotenal or Apocarotenal.**	$C_{30}H_{40}O$ Found inside many plants. It is commercially made from carotene or plants. It is a dark red food color that is soluble in oil. Used in fat based food like margarine, sauces, salad

Color –Red, Orange. Carotene derivative.	dressing, beverages and dairy products such as processed cheese and sweets. No known bad effects listed in sources. Listed for USA, UK, AU, NZ and EU.
E160f **Ethyl ester of Beta-apo-8-cartonoic acid.** Color – Orange. Carotene derivative.	$C_{32}H_{44}O_2$ It is found in small quantities in some plants, and is often commercially produced from apocarotenal (A carotenoid found in spinach and citrus fruits) Used in cheeses. No known bad effects listed in sources. Listed for UK, NZ, AU, and EU. Not listed for USA.
E161 **Xanthophyll.** Color - Yellow.	Made from plants and animals, it is naturally found in green leaves, marigolds and egg yolks. Used in animal feed to color the flesh and to enhance egg yolk color as it is absorbed by the animals and stored in their tissue. No known bad effects indicated in sources. Listed for CAN and USA. Not listed for UK, NZ and AU.
E161a **Flavoxanthin.**	$C_{40}H_{56}O_3$ Flavoxanthin is a xanthophylls (E161), it is industrially made from the Buttercup plant Used very rarely in confectionary. Flavoxanthin is

Color – Golden Yellow.	consumed as part of a normal diet because it is naturally inside many foods. No known bad effects indicated sources. Listed for NZ and AU. Not listed for CAN, USA, EU and UK.
E161b **Lutein.** Color - Golden Yellow.	$C_{40}H_{56}O_2$ Lutein is a natural part of human diet. Found in green leaves, marigolds and egg yolks. It is made commercially from grass or nettles. Lutein is fed to chickens to enhance yolk color. Considered generally safe if used within guidelines. No known bad effects indicated in sources. Listed for NZ, AU, EU, UK. Not listed for CAN and USA.
E161c **Cryptoxanth in.** Color - Yellow.	$C_{40}H_{56}O$ A xanthophyll (E161), made from the Physalis species (part of the nightshade family). It is converted to vitamin A in the human body. Rarely used, sometimes it is inside confectionary. No known bad effects indicated in sources. Listed for NZ, AU and EU. Not listed for UK, CAN and USA.
E161d **Rubixanthin** . Color – Red	$C_{40}H_{56}O$ It is a natural xanthophyll pigment found in many plants. Commercially made from rose hips, considered part of a normal diet. Not available commercially as a food additive so

Orange.	rarely used. No known bad effects indicated in sources. Listed for NZ and AU. Not listed for CAN, UK, EU and USA.
E161e **Violaxanthin.** Color – Orange-Yellow.	$C_{40}H_{56}O_4$ A natural xanthophylls (E161) pigment with an orange color found in a variety of plants including yellow pansies. Not commercially available, and rarely used. No known bad effects indicated in sources. Listed for NZ and AU. Not listed for CAN, USA, EU and UK.
E161f **Rhodoxanthin.** Color – Purple.	$C_{40}H_{50}O_2$ A xanthophylls (E161) pigment with a purple color that is found in small quantities in a variety of plants including *Taxus baccata* (An evergreen tree). Not commercially available and rarely used. No known bad effects indicated in sources. Listed for NZ and AU. Not listed for CAN, USA, EU and UK.
E161g **Canthaxanthin.** Color – Yellow to Orange to Red.	$C_{40}H_{52}O_2$ In nature it is a natural color and food in many plants and animals. Commercially it is made synthetically from carotene. Used in many foods as coloring such as jelly, candy, and breadcrumbs. It is also used to enhance the color of meat and trout and salmon. May cause inability to see at night and aplastic

	anemia (a condition where bone marrow does not produce sufficient new blood cells), has caused death. Listed for CAN, USA and UK. Not listed for AU and NZ.
E162 **Beetroot Red / Betanin.** Color – Red.	$C_{24}H_{27}N_2O_{13}$ A red glycosidic food dye obtained from beets, usually obtained from the extract of beet juice and pulp, source plant may be genetically modified. Used in soup, tomato products, bacon products, desserts, sauces, jams, sweets, jellies. It may be unsuitable for infants and children due to trace amounts of sodium nitrate. No known bad effects in general. Anyone with adverse reaction to beets may need to avoid. Listed for CAN, NZ, AU, UK, USA and EU.
E163 **Anthocyanins.** Color – Red, Purple, Blue.	$C_{21}H_{21}ClO_{10}$ Many colors, red, blue or violet plant pigments present in the cell sap of many flowers, fruits and vegetables. Used in multiple products including soft drinks, pickles, soups, dairy products, jelly, fruit desserts, sweets. No bad effects in general, but caution for asthmatics. Listed for CAN, UK, EU, NZ and AU. Not listed for USA.
E164 **Saffron or**	$C_{44}H_{64}O_{24}$ – Crocin Crocin is the chemical ingredient primarily responsible for the color of

Crocetin or Crocin. Color – Yellow to orange to red.	saffron. Saffron is made from the dried flower and stigma of the saffron crocus flower. The stigma produces the Saffron spice and is red in color. Iran now produces about 90% of world's production of the spice Saffron. Saffron is used in many Asian foods. No known bad effects indicated in sources. Listed for CAN, USA, NZ and AU. Not listed for UK and EU.
E170 **Calcium Carbonate (Chalk).** Color - White Inorganic. Used as a Supplement.	$CaCO_3$ Calcium carbonate is found in rocks and makes up the hard shells of marine life. It is the active ingredient in agricultural lime, and is usually the main cause of hard water. Used in many products including biscuits, sweets, bread, cakes, tinned fruit and vegetables, toothpaste, to firm up canned fruit, in antiacid tablets and calcium supplements. If it is derived from rock mineral or animal bones it can be toxic at really high doses. Caution with taking non plant based supplements long term, and taking any single mineral at high doses long term, as this may throw the body out of balance. No known bad effects listed in sources with proper usage. Listed for CAN, AU, NZ, EU, UK and USA.
E171	TiO_2

Titanium Dioxide or Titanium White or Pigment White 6 or CI 77891. Color – White Inorganic.	Dioxide of Titanium, used in many products for its white color or for its visually clear properties (opacity). Considered chemically inert. Used in horseradish cream and sauces, cottage and Mozzarella cheeses, sweets, toothpaste, sunscreen and white paint. It pollutes waterways and its dust is harmful to lungs. No known bad effects listed in sources for proper additive usage. Listed for USA, CAN, UK, EU, NZ and AU.
E172 **Iron Oxides or Hydroxides.** Color – Red, Yellow, Orange, Brown, Black.	Fe_2O_3 There are many possible molecular forms of iron, all are natural minerals that are commercially made from pure iron powder which create yellow, red, orange, brown or black colors. Some iron is needed in the diet, natural iron as usually eaten in nature is bound up in an plant or animal matrix. Used in salmon and shrimp pastes, desserts and soups. Toxic at high doses and cause kidney damage. Suspected neurotoxin, it also caused blindness in dog studies. Suggest caution and avoid high amounts. Listed for CAN, UK, NZ, EU, AU and USA.
E173 **Aluminum.**	Al Third most abundant element in the earth's crust; 8% by weight. Aluminum metal is too reactive

Color – Grey/Silver Inorganic.	chemically to occur naturally in pure form. Instead, it is found combined with over 270 different minerals The most useful ore of aluminum is bauxite. Aluminum is used in cake decorations, and to add a silvery finish to tablets and pills. It can also be added to water in some areas to make the water clearer and also in some antacid treatments or pills. Despite its prevalence in the environment, aluminum salts are not known to be used by any form of life. There is a lot of aluminum exposure from natural sources. Scientific research is officially unclear at the moment about long term effects when ingesting artificial man made sources of aluminum in normal living. But many people strongly suspect it causes or aggravates health problems such as senility, poor memory, kidney problems, neurological problems, mouth ulcers, mineral malabsoption or mineral imbalances especially in sensitive people with long periods of exposure. The most important consideration is not ingesting too much manmade aluminum. Roughly no more than 1 mg/kg/ per week. Caution with hidden daily sources of aluminum that may add up, like

	excessive antacid usage with aluminum inside it, or using old soft metal aluminum cookware. Need more study. Listed for NZ, USA, CAN, UK, EU, and AU.
E174 **Silver.** Color – Silver Inorganic.	Ag Silver has the highest electrical conductivity of any element and the highest thermal conductivity of any metal. Used rarely in foods as an additive and is usually used for decorating sugar-coated flour sweets. Medicinally silver is an old treatment for infection and illness due to bacteria or viruses etc. Historically considered to be valuable, and safe in medical usage, but has come under attack in recent years. A common use in past times is to put some silver in a jar of milk or water or wine to keep it from spoiling. Silver in colloidal form is used to treat various illnesses. Silver itself is not considered to be toxic, but its salts may be toxic and may build up inside body. This subject needs more objective non bias study as both sides of the silver issue may have conflict of interest. Correctly made colloidal silver is an inexpensive effective treatment for illnesses. Caution with excessive usage. Not listed for USA. Listed for CAN, UK, NZ, AU and EU.

E175 **Gold.** Color –Gold Inorganic.	Au When eaten gold will pass through system; but large amounts may be toxic??(I am not sure how, no clear information on toxic aspect?) Gold has been in use for tooth fillings since the 1800's. Gold is a non reactive metal and very stable and should just pass through the body undigested (Gold is the most stable commonly known substance). Any kind of gold salt or gold compound is another chemical and may be toxic or medicinal. Common usage of gold on food is for surface decoration. Listed for CAN, NZ, AU, UK and EU. Not listed for USA.
E180 **Pigment Rubine Lithol Rubine BK.** Color – Red Inorganic.	$C_{18}H_{12}CaN_2O_6S$ It is a reddish synthetic azo dye, possibly used for coloring cheese rind. Can cause rashes, hives, hyperactivity, stuffy nose, and potentially dangerous to asthmatics. Not listed for CAN, EU, NZ, AU, USA and UK.
E181 **Tannic acid or Tannins.** Clarifying	$C_{76}H_{52}O_{46}$ Derived from the nutgalls and twigs of oak trees or Sicilian Sumac leaves. Safe enough except in high dosages, then gastric problems, possible kidney damage especially excessive amounts over long periods. (Side

agent.	note. Tea contains tannins, which are similar to tannic acid. Depending on individual genetics long term drinking of non herbal tea at high amounts may harm kidneys, by developing painful crystals from the tannins and oxalate. This can cause lower back pain in the kidneys that may be intermixed with other sources of back pain in the lower area of the back. Listed for USA, CAN, AU, NZ and EU. Not listed for UK.

Preservatives E200-E290:

A food preservative is either a natural or synthetic chemical that is added to foods or pharmaceuticals to slow down spoilage, whether from bacterial growth, or undesirable chemical changes. Toxins from bacteria are the live bacteria and their feces and even their dead bodies.

There are many natural kinds of food preservatives such as salt, sugar and vinegar in use in pickling processes. Other kinds of preservatives, especially those made synthetically may be toxic. A longer human history with some of the natural preservatives indicates they may be safer.

E200 **Sorbic Acid.** **(Foods**	$C_6H_8O_2$ Naturally found in fruit, it inhibits fungal growth, but allows bacterial activity. Made from the berries of mountain ash or synthesized from

labeled E200, sometimes may actually contain E201, E202, or E203). Preservatives – Sorbic Acid and its salts.	ketene, an organic compound, sorbic acid is usually put in a salt form where it is most useful and soluble in water. It is used in wine, cheese, fermented products, dried fruits, desert sauces and fillings, soups, sweets, drinks, yeast goods and many others. Listed sources consider it generally safe for most people if ingested occasionally in trace amounts, it is best to avoid excessive use. Sensitive people may have headaches, rashes, skin irritation, hyperactivity, liver problems, intestine upset, and it is a possible mutagen. Choose organic foods to limit or avoid. Listed for USA, AU, UK and EU. Not listed for CAN.
E201 **Sodium sorbate.** Preservative – Sorbic Acid and its salts.	$C_6H_7NaO_2$ Sodium salt of sorbic acid. The main difference between salts of sorbic acid is the different solubility levels. See E200. Listed for CAN, NZ, AU and USA. Not listed for UK and EU.
E202 **Potassium Sorbate.** Preservative – Sorbic Acid	$C_6H_7KO_2$ The potassium salt of sorbic acid. The main difference between salts of sorbic acid is the different solubility levels See E200. Listed for CAN, USA, AU, NZ, UK and EU.

and its salts	
E203 **Calcium Sorbate.** Preservative – Sorbic Acid and its salts.	$C_{12}H_{14}CaO_4$ The calcium salt of sorbic acid. The main difference between salts of sorbic acid is the different solubility levels. Calcium Sorbate is mostly used in dairy products and rye bread. See E200. Listed for CAN, USA, AU, NZ, UK and EU.
E209 **Heptylparaben or (Heptyl para-hydroxybenzoate).** Preservative.	$C_{14}H_{20}O_3$ Found naturally in many foods, especially fruits. Commercially it is synthetically made from toluene, which is then esterified. Used in acidity products such as soft drinks, cordials, sports drinks, salad dressings, condiments, fish, fruit juice concentrates, ciders, vinegar, sauces. May cause or aggravate hyperactivity, skin irritations and behavioral problems in children. Caution for people with asthma or people sensitive to Benzoates. Not listed for AU, NZ, CAN, UK and EU. Listed for USA.
Preservatives made from Benzoic Acid. These are approved for use in most countries.	
E210 **Benzoic Acid.** Preservative -	$C_7H_6O_2$ Found naturally in many foods especially in fruits. Originally made from Benzoin, a resin exuded by trees native to Asia. Made commercially by partial oxidation of toluene with

Benzoic Acid and its salts.	oxygen. Used in alcoholic beverages, baked goods, cheeses, gum, condiments, frozen dairy, relishes, soft sweets, cordials and sugar substitutes. Used in cosmetics as an antiseptic, inside many cough medications and is an antifungal in ointments. Can cause headaches, intestine upset, may increase hyperactivity in affected children. Asthmatics sometimes react badly, may cause asthma attack, especially in those dependant on steroid asthma medications May react to vitamin C in foods or drinks in sunlight to create benzene, a carcinogenic substance. Benzene also can cause cellar death. Often used in concentrations below one percent, which may be lower than required to be labeled. Typical levels of use for Benzoic Acid as a preservative is between 0.05–0.1 percent. Listed for CAN, USA, UK, EU, NZ and AU.
E211 **Sodium Benzoate.** Preservative - Benzoic Acid and its salts.	$NaC_6H_5CO_2$ The sodium salt of Benzoic Acid. It is used to improve the taste of poor food or beverages, for instance orange diet soft drinks may contain a large amount of it, up to 25mg per 250ml. It is also in milk and meat products, relishes and condiments,

	baked goods and, tooth pastes, mouth washes, maple syrup and margarine. It is used in medications including Actifed, Phenergan and Tylenol. Related to Benzoic Acid, see E210. Asthmatics should avoid, it may cause nettle rash, behavioral problems, and hyperactivity. Listed for USA, UK, CAN, EU, NZ and AU.
E212 **Potassium Benzoate.** Preservative - Benzoic Acid and its salts.	$C_7H_5KO_2$ The potassium salt of Benzoic Acid. It can be found in most anything including fruit drinks, pickles, and soft drinks. Related to Benzoic Acid, see E210. Asthmatics should avoid, may cause nettle rash, behavioral problems, hyperactivity. Listed for CAN, UK, USA, EU, NZ and AU.
E213 **Calcium Benzoate.** Preservative - Benzoic Acid and its salts.	$Ca(C_7H_5O_2)_2$ The calcium salt of Benzoic Acid. Typical products include margarine, pickles, fruit juice and many others. Related to Benzoic Acid, see E210. Asthmatics should avoid, it may cause nettle rash, behavioral problems, hyperactivity. Listed for UK, USA, EU, NZ and AU. Not listed for CAN.
E214 **Ethylparabe n,** **(Ethyl para-**	$C_9H_{10}O_3$ It has anesthetic properties and may cause mouth numbness. Typical products include beer, fruit preserves and juices, sauces, syrups, fruit

hydroxyben zoate). Preservative - Benzoic Acid and its salts.	deserts and processed fish. Related to Benzoic Acid, see E210. Asthmatics should avoid, it may cause nettle rash, behavioral problems and hyperactivity. Listed for EU and UK. Not listed for NZ, CAN, USA and AU.
E215 **Sodium ethyl para-hydroxyben zoate, (Sodium Salt of ethyl para-hydroxyben zoate).** Preservative - Benzoic Acid and its salts.	It can be found in shampoos, moisturizers, shaving gels, personal lubricants, spray tanning solution, make up and toothpaste, also used in food as an additive. Related to Benzoic Acid, see E210. Asthmatics should avoid, it may cause nettle rash, behavioral problems and hyperactivity. Listed for EU and UK. Not listed for CAN, USA, NZ and AU.
E216 **Propylparab en, (propyl para-hydroxyben zoate).** Preservative - Benzoic Acid	$C_{10}H_{12}O_3$ Propyl ester of *p*-hydroxybenzoic acid, occurs as a natural substance found in many plants and some insects. It is manufactured synthetically for use in cosmetics, pharmaceuticals and foods. It has anesthetic properties and may cause mouth numbness in concentration. Typical products include beer, fruit preserves and juices, sauces, syrups,

and its salts.	fruit deserts, processed fish. Used in creams, lotions, shampoos and bath products. Asthmatics should avoid, it may cause contact inflammation of the skin, eczema, and mouth numbing in sensitive people. May cause or aggravate hyperactivity and behavioral problems in children. Listed for NZ, AU and CAN. Not listed for USA, UK and EU.
E217 **Sodium propyl para-hydroxyben zoate.** Preservative - Benzoic Acid and its salts.	The sodium salt of propylparaben E216. It is used as a food preservative. Used in water-based cosmetics, such as creams, lotions, shampoos and bath products. Asthmatics should avoid, it may cause contact inflammation of the skin, eczema and mouth numbing in sensitive people. It may cause or aggravate hyperactivity and behavioral problems in children. Listed for CAN. Not listed for UK, NZ, AU and USA.
E218 **Methylpara ben, (Methyl para-hydroxyben zoate).** Preservative -	$C_8H_8O_3$ It is used in a variety of cosmetics and personal care products. Some studies indicate that it safe, but there is mixed information as some sensitive people experience allergic reactions, mainly on the skin, and in the mouth. Listed for NZ, CAN, UK, EU and AU. Not listed for USA.

Benzoic Acid and its salts.	
E219 **Sodium methyl para-hydroxyben zoate.** Preservative - Benzoic Acid and its salts.	The sodium salt of E218, synthesized from Benzoic Acid, it is an anti fungal agent which may be an irritant to the skin and mouth. Listed for EU and UK. Not listed for NZ, CAN, USA and AU.
Sulfur Dioxide and derivatives.	
E220 **Sulphur Dioxide.** Preservative - Sulfur Dioxide and its salts.	SO_2 Derived from coal tar; all sulfur additives are toxic and restricted in use (In the USA, the FDA prohibits their use on raw fruits and vegetables), known to provoke gastric irritation, nausea, headaches, diarrhea, skin rash and asthma attack. Hard to metabolize for those with kidney problems, should be avoided by anyone suffering from conjunctivitis, bronchitis, emphysema, bronchial asthma, or cardiovascular disease. Used in beer, soft drinks, dried fruit, juices, cordials, wine, vinegar, potato products etc. Potato products are a common source of sulfites. Very low concentrations below 10 ppm may

	not be required to be listed on product label--the situation in USA. Sensitive people may be effected by trace amounts. Sulfite intake may be related to increased levels of asthma. Similar adverse properties are possible by all sulfites (E221-E227). Listed for NZ, CAN, EU, UK, AU and USA.
E221 **Sodium Sulfite.** Preservative - Sulfur Dioxide and its salts.	Na_2SO_3 The sodium salt of sulfurous acid. It is a product of sulfur dioxide scrubbing, a part of the flue gas desulphurization process. Typically used in beer, wine, cider, juice, fresh fruit and vegetables, frozen shellfish, jams and pickles etc. Similar as E220, see E220. Listed for CAN, EU, UK, NZ, AU and USA.
E222 **Sodium Hydrogen Sulphite.** Preservative - Sulfur Dioxide and its salts.	$NaHSO_3$ A salt of bisulfate that can be prepared by bubbling sulfur dioxide through a solution of sodium in water. Typically used in beer, wine, cider, juice, fresh fruit and vegetables, frozen shellfish, jams and pickles etc. Similar as E220, see E220. Listed for USA, UK, AU, NZ and EU. Not listed for CAN.
E223 **Sodium Mctabisulph**	$Na_2S_2O_5$. A salt of sulfurous acid. Typically used in beer, wine, cider, juice, fresh fruit and vegetables, frozen shellfish,

ite, Ppyrosulph urous acid, Disodium salt. Preservative - Sulfur Dioxide and its salts.	jams and pickles etc. Used as a bleaching agent in flour. The acceptable daily intake is up to 0.7 mg per kg of body weight. Similar as E220, see E220. Listed for CAN, UK, USA, EU, NZ and AU.
E224 **Potassium Metabisulph ite, Potassium pyrosulfite, Pyrosulfuro us acid dipotassium salt.** Preservative - Sulfur Dioxide and its salts.	$K_2O_5S_2$ A salt of sulfuric acid. It is a preferred condiment sometimes as it does not add sodium to the diet. Typically used in beer, wine, cider, juice, fresh fruit and vegetables, frozen shellfish, jams and pickles etc. Similar as E220, see E220. Listed for CAN, USA, UK, EU, NZ and AU.
E225 **Potassium sulfite.** Preservative - Sulfur Dioxide and its salts.	K_2SO_3 A potassium salt of sulfuric acid. Used in wine, beer, soft drinks, dried fruit, fruit drinks, vinegar, potato products, processed fruits, vegetables, fish, shellfish, deli meats, and others. Similar as E220, see E220. Listed for CAN, AU, NZ and USA. Not listed for UK.

E226 Calcium Sulfite Preservative - Sulfur Dioxide and its salts.	$CaSO_3$ A calcium salt of sulfuric acid. Used as a preservative and firming agent for canned foods etc. Typically used in beer, wine, cider, juice, fresh fruit and vegetables, frozen shellfish, jams and pickles etc. Similar as E220, see E220. Listed for CAN, EU, and UK. Not listed for NZ, AU and USA.
E227 Calcium Hydrogen Sulfite. Preservative - Sulfur Dioxide and its salts.	$Ca(HSO_3)_2$ A salt of sulfuric acid. Preservative and firming agent for canned foods. Typically used in beer, wine, cider, juice, fresh fruit and vegetables, frozen shellfish, jams and pickles etc. Similar as E220, see E220. Listed for EU and UK. Not listed for NZ, CAN, AU and USA.
E228 Potassium Bisulfite Preservative - Sulfur Dioxide and its salts.	$KHSO_3$. Preservative and firming agent for canned foods. It is used during the production of alcoholic beverages as a sterilizing agent. Typically used in beer, wine, cider, juice, fresh fruit and vegetables, frozen shellfish, jams and pickles etc. Similar as E220, see E220. Listed for CAN, USA, UK, AU, NZ and EU.
Biphenyl, and others.	
E230 Biphenyl, Diphenyl.	$C_{12}H_{10}$ Made from benzene, it is an anti-fungal substance used as a prescrvative to prevent the growth of

Preservative - Biphenyl and its derivatives.	molds, and fungi on citrus fruit during shipment, transportation and storage. Sometimes one can notice a unknown film on treated fruit which may cause a bad reaction. It is a fungicide used for waxing citrus fruits. Wash all fruit with soapy brush and buy organic when you can. Factory workers exposed sometimes have a bad reaction, including headache, nausea, gastrointestinal pain, vomiting, indigestion, numbness, aching of limbs, eyes and respiratory tract irritation, and general fatigue, may be carcinogenic. Listed for USA, UK and EU. Not listed for CAN, NZ and AU.
E231 **Orthopheny l phenol or 2-Phenylphen ol.** **Other names.** Remol TRF or Preventol O Extra or Orthoxenol, Ortho-	$C_{12}H_{10}O$ It is an organic compound that consists of two linked benzene rings and a phenolic hydroxyl group. Typically used on fruit such as pears, carrots, peaches, plums, prunes, sweet potato, pineapples, tomatoes, peppers, cherries and nectarines. It is a fungicide used for waxing citrus fruits. Wash all fruit with soapy brush and buy organic. Sometimes one can notice a glossy oily film on treated fruit that may cause a bad reaction. It may be in household goods, for instance in a spray disinfectant, or in underarm

Hydroxydiphenyl or Ortho-Hydroxybiphenylortho or Ortho-Diphenylol or Ortho-Biphenylol Dowicide 1 or 2-Hydroxydiphenyl or 2-Hydroxybiphenyl. Preservative - Biphenyl and its derivatives.	deodorant. It may irritate eyes and skin, can be carcinogenic and a mutant causing agent. Listed for EU. Not listed for UK, CAN, AU, NZ and USA.
E232 **Sodium Biphenyl-2-yl Oxide.** Preservative - Biphenyl and its derivatives.	$C_{12}H_9NaO$ It is the sodium salt of 2-phenylphenol. Typically used on fruit such as pears, carrots, peaches, plums, prunes, sweet potato, pineapples, tomatoes, peppers, cherries, nectarines. It is a fungicide used for waxing citrus fruits. Wash all fruit with soapy brush and buy organic. Sometimes one can notice a film on treated fruit that may cause a bad reaction. It may be a cancer mutation agent and a skin or eye irritant. See E231. Listed for USA and EU. Not listed for UK, CAN, NZ and

	AU.
E233 **Thiabendaz ole** **or** **Tiabendazol e** **or** **TBZ.** **Trade names, Mintezol, Tresaderm, Arbotect.** Preservative – other.	$C_{10}H_7N_3S$ Used to protect fruits during storage and shipping. Typically used on fruit such as pears, carrots, peaches, plums, prunes, sweet potato, pineapples, tomatoes, peppers, cherries and nectarines. It can be used in conjunction with wax on fruits. Wash all fruit with soapy brush and buy organic. Sometimes one can notice a film on treated fruit that may cause a bad reaction. It is antiparasitic and can help control roundworms or hookworms etc. It is a chelating agent, which means that it is used medicinally to bind metals in metal poisoning cases, such as lead poisoning, mercury poisoning or antimony poisoning. For human drug usage it has serious negative side effects. In dogs and cats it is used to treat ear infections. Not super toxic in proper usage on fruits but best to scrub it off. Not listed for UK, CAN, AU, NZ, USA and EU.
E234 **Nisin** Antibiotic derived from bacteria,	$C_{143}H_{230}N_{42}O_{37}S_7$ Broad spectrum antibiotic made from the bacterium Lactococcus lactis. It is used as a preservative against bacteria. Used in beer, processed cheese products, tomato paste, dairy products, canned food,

Preservative.	baked foods and many others. In foods, it is common to use Nisin at levels ranging from ~1-25ppm; listed sources indicate it is safe in proper usage. Listed for USA, AU, NZ, UK and EU. Not listed for CAN.
E235 **Natamycin or Pimaracin.** Mould inhibitor.	$C_{33}H_{47}NO_{13}$ A naturally occurring antifungal agent produced during fermentation by the bacterium *Streptomyces natalensis*, commonly found in soil. It is sometimes used medically to treat candidiasis, when so it may cause nausea, vomiting anorexia, diarrhea and skin irritation. Typical products are meat, cheese, cottage cheese, sour cream and yogurt. In humans, a dose of 500 mg/kg/day (a very high dosage as compared to its proper usage in food) repeated over multiple days' causes nausea, vomiting, and diarrhea. Caution for sensitive people as a food additive. Listed for CAN, UK, EU, USA, NZ and AU.
E236 **Formic acid or Formylic acid.** Preservative.	CH_2O_2 It is naturally found in the stings and bites of many insects also in stinging nettle. It is industrially synthesized from carbon monoxide. Used in food as a preservative and anti bacterial agent, soluble in water and has diuretic properties. Used in sauces,

	gravies, dressings, drinks, and baked goods. Can cause kidney damage with excessive ingestion, and nausea, vomiting, diarrhea and skin irritation. Listed for USA. Not listed for NZ, CAN, UK, AU and EU.
E237 **Sodium formate or Formic acid sodium salt.** Preservative or diuretic.	HCOONa It is the sodium salt of Formic acid E236. Used in several fabric dyeing and printing processes. Also used in sauces, gravies, dressings, drinks, and baked goods. A diuretic in high concentration. See E236. Listed for USA. Not listed for CAN, UK, AU, NZ and EU.
E238 **Calcium formate.** Preservative or diuretic.	$Ca(HCOO)_2$ It is the calcium salt of Formic acid E236. Can be made synthetically by reacting calcium oxide or calcium hydroxide with formic acid. Used in sauces, gravies, dressings, drinks, and baked goods. A diuretic in high concentration. See E236. Not listed for UK, NZ, USA, CAN, AU and EU.
E239 **Hexamine.** Preservative.	$C_6H_{12}N_4$ It is made by the reaction of formaldehyde and ammonia. It is used in sauces, gravies, dressings, drinks, and baked goods. Can be used as medication in urinary tract infections, but caution with overtaxing the kidneys. May cause

	skin disorders, rashes, stomach upset and cancer. Listed for EU and UK. Not listed for CAN, USA, NZ and AU.
E240 **Formaldehy de** **Other names: formalin, formic aldehyde, methylene oxide, oxomethane , paraform.** Preservative.	CH_2O It is commercially made with methanol. Naturally in smoked meats, rarely put on foods, but used in cosmetics. It is very toxic by inhalation, ingestion and through skin absorption-it may cause burns. A cancer hazard, mutagen, can damage kidneys, may cause allergic reactions, can be absorbed through skin. May cause heritable genetic damage to offspring. Very destructive of mucous membranes, upper respiratory tract and eyes and skin, causing eye tearing, headaches, sinus congestion etc. It is inside many building and bedding products, in foam bedding, a extreme danger to infants. It is especially concentrated in new products, it may be better to used aged construction or bedding products or better yet use clean natural products. Listed for USA. Not listed for CAN, UK, NZ, AU and EU.
E242 **Dimethyl dicarbonate or DMDC.**	$C_4H_6O_5$ It is a yeast inhibitor and preservative. Used in fruit drinks, sport drinks, beer and wine. Considered safe as it breaks down in the liquid, with no traces of toxin in

Dimethyl Pyrocarbonate Preservative	the final product. Listed sources regard it as safe in proper usage. Listed for EU, UK, NZ, AU and USA. Not listed for CAN.
Nitrates	
E249 **Potassium Nitrate.** Preservative - mainly for meats.	KNO_2 It is a color fixative and curing agent for meat. Used in processed and cured meats, such as bacon, sausage, ham, hot dogs, salami, smoked and cured fish. Nitrites in concentration may effect the body's ability to carry oxygen, resulting in shortness of breath, dizziness and headaches, feeling of illness; cancer causing. Over time can build up inside the body and organs causing cancer and disease, it may cause colon cancer and other organ cancers. Extra caution if eating a lot of processed meats. Not permitted in foods for infants and young children. Listed for CAN, USA, UK, EU, NZ and AU.
E250 **Sodium Nitrite.** Preservative - mainly for meats.	$NaNO_2$ It is a color fixative and curing agent for meat. Used in processed and cured meats, such as bacon, sausage, ham, hot dogs, salami, smoked and cured fish. Nitrites in concentration may effect the body's ability to carry oxygen, resulting in shortness of breath, dizziness and headaches,

	feeling of illness. It is cancer causing. Over time can build up inside the body and organs causing cancer and disease, it may cause colon cancer and other organ cancers. Extra caution if eating a lot of processed meats. Not permitted in foods for infants and young children. Listed for CAN, USA, UK, NZ, EU and AU.
E251 **Sodium Nitrate or Chile saltpeter or Cubic nitre or Nitric acid sodium salt**. Preservative - mainly for meats.	$NaNO_3$ It is a natural mineral, also known as *Chile saltpeter* or *Peru saltpeter* (due to the large deposits found in each country), it can be made synthetically. Used in processed and cured meats, such as bacon, sausages, ham, hot dogs, salami, smoked and cured fish. May provoke hyperactivity and other adverse reactions, carcinogenic, may build up in body and cause colon cancer and other organ cancers. Extra caution if eating a lot of processed meats. Not permitted in foods for infants and young children. Listed for CAN, USA, UK, AU, NZ and EU.
E252 **Potassium Nitrate (Saltpeter).** Preservative -	KNO_3 It is an ionic salt of potassium ions K^+ and nitrate ions NO_3^-. Used in processed and cured meats, such as bacon, sausages, ham, hot dogs, salami, smoked and cured fish. It may cause hyperactivity, behavioral

mainly for meats.	problems in children, asthma, headaches, dizziness, and kidney problems, it may build up in body. May cause colon cancer and other organ cancers. Extra caution if eating a lot of processed meats. Prohibited in foods for infants and young children. Listed for CAN, USA, UK, AU, NZ and EU.
Miscellaneous acids and their salts.	
E260 Acetic Acid Miscellaneous - Acids and their Salts Acidity regulator Preservative Anti-microbial Flavor enhancer	$C_2H_4O_2$ It is naturally found in vinegar, Used to acidify food as a preservative and for flavoring. About 10% of world production is made by bacteria action and 75% by methanol carbonylation as some countries require Acetic Acid from a natural source. May cause gastric distress, and eye, skin irritation. Used in condiments, pickled vegetables, sauces, snack foods, bread, cake, dressings, seasonings, baked foods, wines, soups and noodle products etc. Vinegar is typically 4-18% acetic acid by mass. Concentrated acetic acid is strong and dangerous. Considered safe in normal food usage in listed sources, but I wonder about the chemically made product. Listed for CAN, AU, NZ, UK, USA and EU.
E261	CH_3CO_2K It is a potassium salt of acetic acid

Potassium Acetate, or Acetic acid potassium salt or Potassium ethanoate or Ethanoic acid potassium salt. Acidity regulator Preservative Anti-microbial Flavor enhancer	see E260, a preservative and acidity regulator. Used in condiments, pickled vegetables, sauces, snack foods, bread, cake, dressings, seasonings, baked foods, wines, soups and noodle products etc. It may cause headaches and intestine upset, it should be avoided by people with impaired kidneys or liver. Typical products are sauces and pickles. Listed for UK, USA, AU, NZ, EU and NZ. Not listed for CAN.
E262 **Sodium acetate and Sodium diacetate.** Acidity regulator Preservative Anti-microbial	Sodium acetate -$C_2H_3NaO_2$, Sodium diacetate- $NaC_4H_7O_4$ They are a sodium salt of acetic acid, see E260. As a acidity regulator they may be part of flavoring of artificial salt and vinegar potato chips. Mold inhibitor in snack foods and bread, flavor enhancer in breads, cakes, cheese and snack foods etc. Both have no known adverse affects in listed sources. Listed for UK, USA, EU, NZ, AU and CAN.

Flavor enhancer	
E263 **Calcium Acetate or Calcium acetate or monohydrate or Calcium diacetate.** Acidity regulator Preservative Anti-microbial Flavor enhancer	$Ca(OAc)_2$ It is the calcium salt of acetic acid. Used as a thickening agent and buffer in controlling the pH of food during processing, as a preservative to prevent microbial growth, and as a calcium supplement in pet products. Used in cake mixtures, breads, puddings, soups, wines, pie fillings and candies etc. May cause eye, skin, respiratory irritation. Listed for UK, CAN, NZ, AU, EU and USA.
E264 **Ammonium acetate.** Acidity regulator Preservative Anti-microbial Flavor enhancer	$C_2H_3O_2NH_4$ It is made from the reaction of ammonia and acetic acid. Used in products that contains acetates, such as in cake mixtures, breads, puddings, soups, wines, pie fillings and candies etc. May cause nausea and vomiting in sensitive people. Excess ammonia is toxic, but it is naturally inside the body because it is a product of protein catabolism and is safely removed by the by the liver. Normal blood ammonia levels range

	from 10-40 µmol/L. This may increase by 10% with exposure to 25 ppm, but is not considered harmful for most people. People with liver dysfunction may be at increased risk for ammonia toxicity. Early symptoms of ammonia toxicity related to decreasing liver function include inability to concentrate, sleepiness and being prone to irritability. Listed for NZ, AU and USA. Not listed for UK, EU and CAN.
E265 **Dehydroace tic acid** Acidity regulator Preservative Anti-microbial Flavor enhancer	$C_8H_8O_4$ Used mostly as a fungicide and bactericide. It is used to reduce pickle bloating, as a preservative for squash and strawberries. In high concentrations it may be toxic to kidneys, liver and a skin irritant. It is effective against bacteria and fungi at low concentrations. It is used in a wide variety of products including sunscreens, skin care, cosmetics, bath, fragrance, shaving, hair care, nail care and eye and facial makeup. Listed for USA. Not listed for UK, NZ, AU, CAN and EU.
E266 **Sodium Dehydroace tate.**	$C_8H_7NaO_4$ It is the sodium salt of dehydroacetic acid, see E265. Used mostly as a fungicide and bactericide. It is used to reduce pickle bloating, as a preservative for squash and

Acidity regulator Preservative Anti-microbial Flavor enhancer	strawberries. In high concentrations it may be toxic to kidneys, liver and a skin irritant. It is effective against bacteria and fungi at low concentrations. It is used in a wide variety of products including sunscreens, skin care, cosmetics, bath, fragrance, shaving, hair care, nail care and eye and facial makeup. Listed for USA. Not listed for UK, NZ, AU, CAN and EU.
E270 **Lactic acid or Milk acid** Acidity regulator Preservative Anti-microbial Flavor enhancer	$C_3H_6O_3$ It is a food acid produced by heating and fermenting carbohydrates in milk whey, potatoes, cornstarch or molasses (these may be genetically modified). It is hard for babies to metabolize as they have not yet developed the appropriate enzymes in the liver to metabolize these forms of lactate. Used in sweets, dressings, soft drinks and may be in beer, also may be in infant formulas. Although the name refers to milk, it may be not made from milk and thus possibly suitable for people with milk allergy or lactose intolerance. Listed for UK, NZ, AU, EU, USA and CAN.
E280 **Propionic Acid or**	$C_3H_6O_2$ It is mostly commercially produced by the hydrocarboxylation of ethylene using nickel carbonyl as the catalyst. Propanoic acid inhibits the

Propanoic acid (meaning as from propane). Acidity regulator Preservative Anti-microbial Flavor enhancer. Propionic acid and it's salts, sodium, calcium and potassium Propionates are the main preservatives in breads, bakery goods, and flour products.	growth of mold and some bacteria at the levels between 0.1 and 1% by weight Used in breads, baked goods and flour based products and pizzas, and cheeses. Propionates occur naturally in fermented foods, human perspiration and ruminants digestive tract, also can be derived commercially from ethylene and carbon monoxide or propionaldehyde or natural gas or fermented wood pulp; produced when bacteria decompose fiber; commonly used in cheese, bread and flour products. Most propanoic acid produced is consumed as a preservative for both animal feed and food for human consumption. Any additive less than 1% may not be on the food label. Propionates are thought to be linked with migraine headaches; behavioral and learning problems, headaches and asthma. Listed for UK, CAN, AU, NZ, EU, USA and NZ.
E281 **Sodium Propionate.** Acidity	$C_3H_5NaO_2$ It is the sodium salt of propionic acid, see E280. Used to prevent bacteria, a mold inhibitor and anti fungal agent. It is a mold inhibitor commonly used in bakery products.

regulator, Preservative, Anti-microbial, Flavor enhancer.	It occurs naturally in fermented food, human sweat and the stomachs of cows. Typical products are processed cheese, flour, and bread products. It may irritate eyes and skin, readily absorbed through the skin. May cause migraines, behavioral and learning problems, skin irritation, headaches and asthma. Listed for UK, CAN, AU, USA, EU and NZ.
E282 Calcium Propionate. Acidity regulator, Preservative, Anti-microbial, Flavor enhancer.	$C_6H_{10}CaO_4$ It is the calcium salt of propanoic acid. Calcium propanoate is used in bakery products as a mold inhibitor, typically at 0.1-0.4% (though animal feed may contain up to 1%). Typical products are processed cheese, flour, and bread products, can be used as a fungicide on fruit. May be linked to migraines, behavioral and learning problems, skin irritation, headaches and asthma. See E281. Listed for UK, NZ, AU, USA, EU and CAN.
E283 **Potassium Propionate.** Acidity regulator, Preservative, Anti-microbial,	$C_3H_5KO_2$ It is the potassium salt of propanoic acid. Typical products are processed cheese, flour, and bread products May be linked to migraines, behavioral and learning problems, skin irritation, headaches and asthma. See E281. Listed for UK, NZ, AU, EU and CAN. Not listed for USA.

Flavor enhancer.	
E284 **Boric Acid, or Hydrogen borate or Boracic acid or Orthoboric acid or Acidum boricum.** Acidity regulator, Preservative, Anti-microbial, Flavor enhancer, Insecticide.	H_3BO_3 It is made from borate and sulfuric acid. Used in wood as a preservative for leather finishing, in paints, soaps, and in ceramics and glass manufacturing. Can be used to control ants and cockroaches, suspected to be a toxic hazard to the human nervous system. Ingestion is harmful and may be fatal, harmful by inhalation. An irritant. May cause congenital malformation in the fetus. Classified as toxic for reproduction. Boric acid solutions to be used as an eye wash or on abraded skin are known to be particularly toxic to infants, especially with repeated use, because of their slow elimination rate. Considered safe enough for most adults for very occasional usage as a skin or eye wash with a weak concentration, for instance a 1.5% solution. Continuous ingestion of boric acid in small amounts is toxic, and may cause kidney damage and eventually kidney failure. Rarely used inside foods, no known food additive usages, but may be used illegally in some third world countries. Listed for UK, NZ, AU, EU and USA. Not listed for CAN.

E285	$Na_2B_4O_7 \cdot 10H_2O$
Borax or Borax decahydrate or Boricin or Disodium tetraborate decahydrate . Acidity regulator, Preservative, Anti-microbial, Flavor enhancer. insecticide.	It is a salt of boric acid or sodium tetraborate. Borax is obtained by mining of boron-containing rocks, or by recrystallization from water sources. A major source of borax is the mineral kernite, abundant in the Mojave Desert. It may cause reproductive disorders, based on tests with laboratory animals. It is an eye and skin irritant. Harmful by ingestion, may be harmful by inhalation. Rarely used in foods, no known food additive usages. Not listed for NZ, AU and CAN. Listed for UK, USA and EU.
E290 **Carbon Dioxide.** Preservative, Anti-microbial, Flavor enhancer, Acidity regulator.	CO_2 Propellant, coolant, produced by the action of acidified water on limestone or dolomite, it may increase the effect of alcohol; typical products are wine, soft drinks and confectionary. It is a possible toxic hazard even though it is a natural gas that you breathe out around 2.3 pounds a day. More than 10% concentration in air causes blackouts. In concentration it may cause reproductive problems and is a neurotoxin, a potential

developmental toxin, and has possible links to infertility. Generally considered safe in common usage, but caution with concentrated ingestion(sodas) or inhalation. Listed for UK, CAN, AU, NZ and USA.

Acids, Antioxidants & Salts E296-E385:

Food acids are added to make flavors more tart or strong, and also act as a preservatives and antioxidant. Well known food acids include, vinegar, tartaric acid, malic acid, fumaric acid, lactic acid and citric acid.

Antioxidants such as the vitamin C group act as preservatives by inhibiting the effects of oxygen on food, and as a bonus are often beneficial to health.

E296 **Malic Acid** Acidity regulator, Preservative, Anti-microbial, Flavor enhancer, Sequestrant(binding agent).	$C_4H_6O_5$ It is naturally in fruits. The most is found in green apples. Malic acid contributes to the sourness of green apples. Products include canned fruit, vegetables, jams, jelly, frozen vegetables soups, broths, beer, ciders, vinegars, condiments, sauces, batters, pre-cooked foods and processed meats. A neurotoxin (kills or harms nerve cells), a potential developmental toxin and has possible links to infertility. Infants and young children should avoid it. Listed for UK, CAN, EU, USA, AU and NZ.

E297 Fumaric acid. Acidity regulator, Preservative, Anti-microbial, Flavor enhancer, Raising agent.	$C_4H_4O_4$ It is made by the oxidation of benzene or by bacterial fermentation in glucose. Used in baked foods, breads, fruit juice, wine, confectionary, jams, , pie fillings, gelatin, cake mixes, soft drinks, dry mixes, baking powder, baked goods, dairy products, meat, poultry, eggs and nuts, etc. It is relatively inexpensive and used as a replacement for other more expensive acids. Not much information, no known bad effects noted in sources. Listed for UK, CAN, EU, USA, AU and NZ.
E300 **Ascorbic Acid, Commonly known as Vitamin C.** Antioxidant, Preservative, Acidity regulator, Supplement.	$C_6H_8O_6$ It is synthetically made for commercial usage. Used in many foods and drinks such as, bakery products, sauces, soups and broths, breakfast cereals, vinegars and dressings, meat casings, sports drinks, energy drinks, dairy based products and many others. Essential for health, need daily intake because the human body stores too little of it and can't make it. Used to flavor and acidify foods and as an antioxidant or raising agent. Safe and healthy in moderate daily amounts. Large doses may cause diarrhea, dizziness and kidney stones, long term excessive

	supplementation may cause an imbalance of body minerals. I think it is best to have supplements taken in balance with each other (using a balanced formula) and to use food based supplements, especially when taking supplementation long term. This method helps to prevent imbalances in the body. Listed for UK, USA, CAN, AU, EU and NZ.
E301 **Sodium Ascorbate Other names: Ascorbic acid or Sodium salt or Ascorbicin or Ascorbin or Cebitate or Cenolate or Monosodium Ascorbate.** Antioxidant, Preservative, Acidity regulator.	$C_6H_7NaO_6$ Sodium salt of vitamin C. See E300. Considered generally safe in listed sources. Listed for UK, USA, AU, CAN, EU and NZ.

E302 **Calcium Ascorbate. Acidity regulator Vitamin C and derivatives.** Antioxidant, Preservative.	$C_{12}H_{14}CaO_{12}$ It is the calcium salt of ascorbic acid. Considered generally safe in listed sources. May increase the formation of calcium oxalate stones, meaning making stones in kidney or bladder. See E300. Considered generally safe in listed sources. Listed for UK, USA, AU, EU and NZ
E303 **Potassium Ascorbate. Acidity regulator Vitamin C and derivatives.** Antioxidant, Preservative.	$C_6H_7KO_6$ The potassium salt of ascorbic acid, see E300. Considered generally safe in listed sources. Not listed for UK, CAN, EU and USA. Listed for AU and NZ
E304 **Ascorbyl palmitate. Antioxidant s, Vitamin C and derivatives.**	$C_{22}H_{38}O_7$ Ascorbyl palmitate is an ester formed from ascorbic acid and palmitic acid creating a fat-soluble form of vitamin C. A source of vitamin C, and an antioxidant in food, it has many applications because its soluble in fats at high temperatures. Products include cereal and processed meat

Fatty acid ester of Ascorbic acid.	products. See E300. Considered generally safe in noted sources. Listed for UK, CAN, EU, USA, AU and NZ.
E305 **Ascorbyl stearate. Antioxidants- Vitamin C and derivatives.** Fatty acid ester of Ascorbic acid.	$C_{24}H_{42}O_7$ Ascorbyl stearate is made from both esterification of stearic acid and ascorbic acid together. It is used as a source of vitamin C, and an antioxidant in food. Products include cereal and processed meat products. See E300. Considered generally safe in noted sources. Not listed for UK, AU, NZ and EU. Listed for CAN and USA.
E306 **Tocopherols concentrate, or all "forms" of Vitamin E naturally together in a concentrate.** Antioxidants- Vitamin E.	C28H48O2 Compounds in soya bean oil, wheat germ, rice germ, cottonseed, maize and green leaves are full of naturally occurring vitamin E. It is extracted to be used in food as antioxidants and sources of vitamin enrichment. These tocopherols include alpha-, beta-, gamma- and delta-tocopherols. Vitamin E is an essential vitamin which means the body regularly needs outside sources. Typical products include vegetable oils, meat products, soups, baby formulas, margarine and salad dressings. Considered generally safe in noted sources. Listed for UK, NZ, AU, EU

	and CAN. Not listed for USA.
E307 **Alpha-Tocopherol, Synthetically made Vitamin E.** Antioxidants-Vitamin E.	$C_{29}H_{50}O_2$ It is a chemically synthesized form of vitamin E. Products include vitamin enriched foods, vegetable oils, cheese, soups, processed meat products, margarine and salad dressings Considered generally safe in noted sources, see E306. Listed for NZ, UK, AU, EU and USA. Not listed for CAN.
E308 **Gamma-Tocopherol Synthetically made Vitamin E.** Antioxidants-Vitamin E.	$C_{28}H_{48}O_2$ Chemically synthesized and used as a source of vitamin E. . Products include synthetically vitamin enriched foods, vegetable oils, cheese, soups, processed meat products, margarine and salad dressings. Considered generally safe in listed sources., see 306. Listed for UK, NZ, AU and EU. Not listed for CAN and USA.
E309 **Delta-Tocopherol Synthetically made Vitamin E.** Antioxidants-Vitamin E.	$C_{27}H_{46}O_2$ Chemically synthesized, used as a source of vitamin E. Products include synthetically vitamin enriched foods, vegetable oils, cheese, soups, processed meat products, margarine and salad dressings. Considered generally safe in noted sources, see 306. Listed for UK, NZ, AU and EU. Not listed for CAN and USA.
E310	$C_{10}H_{12}O_5$

Propyl Gallate. Antioxidants-other.	Since 1948 this antioxidant has been added to foods containing oils and fats to prevent oxidation or rancidity. Used in margarines, lard, snack food, and salad dressing. May cause gastric or skin irritation, also may cause allergic reaction. Gallates are not permitted in foods for infants and small children because of their known tendency to cause the blood disorder methemoglobinem. A suspected carcinogen, asthmatics and aspirin sensitive people should avoid, it may cause liver damage and skin irritations. Used in oils, margarine, lard and salad dressings, cosmetics and hair products. It can be used with BHT (E321) and BHA (E320), it is unstable at high temperatures so it has limited range of use in foods. Listed for UK, NZ, AU, EU, CAN and USA.
E311 **Octyl Gallate.** Antioxidants-other.	$C_{15}H_{22}O_5$ It is synthesized by the etherification of gallic acid. Similar too E310, and see E310. Listed for UK, EU, AU, NZ and USA. Not listed for CAN.
E312 Dodecyl Gallate.	$C_{19}H_{30}O_5$ It is synthesized by the etherification of gallic acid. Similar too E310, and see E310. Listed for UK, EU, NZ, AU

Antioxidants-other.	and USA. Not listed for CAN.
E313 **Ethyl gallate,** **or** **Thiodipropionic acid.** Antioxidants-other.	$C_9H_{10}O_5$ It is a synthetic anti-oxidant made as an ester formed by the condensation of gallic acid and ethanol. Found in foods that contain oils and fats such as margarines, lard, salad dressings and cosmetics. Up to 3 mg/kg by weight in foods. No known side effects in the concentrations used. Not much information. Not listed for NZ, UK, AU, EU and CAN. Listed for USA.
E314 **Guaiac Gum.** Antioxidants-other.	It is a natural resin from the tree Guajacum officinale and some related tropical trees. A anti-oxidant in cola products, used in some chewing gums (Japan), in low sugar jams and sauces. Up to 2.5 mg/kg body weight. Normally no bad effects in concentrations used, but some adverse reactions are reported sensitive people. Listed for CAN and USA. Not listed for UK, AU and NZ.
E315 **Erythorbic acid,** **or** **Isoascorbic acid.**	$C_6H_8O_6$ It is made from Sucrose. Since the U.S. Food and Drug Administration banned the use of sulfites as a preservative in foods intended to be eaten fresh (such as salad bar ingredients), the use of erythorbic acid as a food preservative has

Antioxidants-other.	increased. It has the same molecular structure as vitamin C, but has a different three dimensional shape (stereoisomer). It is also used as a preservative in cured meats and frozen vegetables in dairy-based drinks, processed cheeses, fat spreads, processed fruit, canned vegetables, breakfast cereals, sweeteners, vinegars, and mustards. No known adverse effects in sources. Listed for UK, AU, NZ, EU, USA and CAN.
E316 **Sodium erythorbate.** Antioxidants-other.	$C_6H_7NaO_6$ It is the sodium salt of erythorbic acid. It is in greater usage because the food industry has responded to that some people are allergic to sulfites and to the USA ban on sulfites. Sodium erythorbate is produced from sugars derived from different sources, such as beets, sugar cane, and corn, which may be genetically modified. Used in meats such as hot dogs, beef sticks and soft drinks. No know bad effects noted in sources. See E315. Listed for UK, NZ, AU, EU, USA and CAN.
E317 **Erythorbin acid.**	$C_6H_8O_6$ It is a stereoisomer (same molecular formula but different shape) of ascorbic acid (vitamin C), but no vitamin value. Made from Sucrose

Antioxidants-other.	which may be corn based and genetically modified. It is used in frozen fish, preserved meat and fish, processed fruit, canned vegetables, breakfast cereals, sweeteners, and other foods that use ascorbic acid. No known adverse reactions in sources. Not listed for UK, USA, EU, NZ, AU and CAN.
E318

Sodium erythorbate or Sodium Isoascorbate.

Antioxidants-other. | $C_6H_7NaO_6$
The sodium salt of Erythorbic acid. See E317. Used in meats, poultry and soft drinks. No known adverse effects noted in sources. Not listed for NZ, AU, UK and EU. Listed for CAN and USA. |
| **E319**

Tert-Butylhydroquinone (TBHQ).

Antioxidants-other. | $C_{10}H_{14}O_2$
Petroleum based aromatic organic compound which is a type of phenol, and a kind of butane, it can cause nausea, vomiting and delirium. It is linked to cancer and birth defects. A dose of 5g is considered fatal. The highest limit is (1000 mg/kg) permitted for frozen fish and fish products. The FDA sets an upper limit of 0.02% in oil or fat content in foods (so it may not be listed on the ingredients as it is below one |

	percent). It increases storage life. Typical products are dairy, edible fats and oils, margarine, salad dressing, baked goods, salad dressings and lipstick. May be linked to cancer, birth defects, can cause nausea, vomiting, delirium, collapse, and dermatitis with very high dosages. Very few people have noticeable adverse reactions with the acceptable food additive concentrations. It needs more testing for long term effects with concentrations used. Listed for UK, AU, NZ, USA, CAN and EU.
E320 **Butylated Hydroxyani sole (BHA).** Antioxidants-other.	$C_{11}H_{16}O_2$ A petroleum product derivative, BHA is a synthetic molecule similar to vitamin E. Typical products include biscuits, cakes, fats and oils, cereals, pastry products, sweets, edible oils, chewing gum, fats, margarine, nuts, instant potato products and polyethylene food wraps. It is not permitted inside infant foods. May increase hyperactivity in affected children and asthmatics sometimes react badly. Be cautious if you suffer from allergies or intolerances. Be cautious with babies, BHA can be used in baked products because it is stable at high temperatures; it is mainly used to prevent rancidity in

	fats and oils. May provoke an allergic reaction in some people, also may cause hyperactivity and other intolerances and accumulate in body fat. May be carcinogenic and have estrogenic effects. Listed for UK, AU, NZ, EU, CAN and USA.
E321 **Butylated Hydroxytol uene (BHT).** Antioxidants-other.	$C_{15}H_{24}O$ It is a petroleum derivative, BHA is a synthetic molecule similar to vitamin E. See E320 It is one of the most commonly used antioxidants for food oils and fats and is cheaper than BHA, but has more limited use because of being unstable at high temperature. There is evidence that BHT causes cell division (premature ageing). Common products, biscuits, cakes, fats and oils, cereals, pastry, and sweets. Listed for UK, NZ, AU, USA, EU and CAN.
E322 **Lecithin.** Emulsifiers and Stabilizers.	$C_{40}H_{80}NO_8P$ Lecithin is extracted from soy beans, egg yolks and leguminous seeds, corn or animal resources. It is non toxic, used to allow an combination and stable mixture of oils in margarine, chocolate, mayonnaise, milk powder, potato chips, puddings and cereals. It plays an important role in the transmission of nerve impulses. Present in all living cells and is a significant constituent of nerve and

	brain tissues. It is a fat emulsifier therefore it is good for cleaning out clogged arteries, but use carefully to not release too much arterial fat all at once. It helps mental function, and brain power. Those with egg allergy should avoid Lecithin made from eggs. No known bad effects noted in sources. Listed for UK, NZ, AU, USA, EU and CAN.
E323 **Anoxomer.** Anti-oxidant, Preservative.	It is a synthetic non-digestible polymeric antioxidant. It is by design unable to be digested or absorbed by the human body. Used in oils and animal fats, in fish oils, chewing gum, baked products, potato chips, and processed meats. No strong information on safety either way in listed sources, but appears safe at this time. Not listed for UK, EU, NZ and AU. Listed for USA.
E324 **Ethoxyquin.** Anti-oxidant, Preservative.	$C_{14}H_{19}NO$ A quinoline-based antioxidant used as a food preservative and pesticide. Used in pet foods, such as dog foods, no indication of being in human food, but may be? Avoid it, it may cause chronic illnesse and weak health for both humans and pets. Possibly in a concentration less than 1%, so may not be on product label--- often used at 75 parts per million or less. Try to buy natural or whole food

	pet food or organic pet food etc. Or feed pets clean table scraps. Not listed for UK, EU, AU, NZ and CAN. Listed for USA. http://www.holisticvetpetcare.com/ethoxyquin.htm
E325 **Sodium Lactate.** (Miscellaneous - Salts of Lactic Acid). Preservative, Acidity regulator.	$C_3H_5NaO_3$ It is a sodium salt of lactic acid, see E270. Made by fermentation of a sugar source, such as corn or beets (these may be genetically modified), and then neutralizing the resulting lactic acid. Usually no adverse reactions for adults. (Its name sounds similar to milk sugar, lactose, but it is totally different.) Small children and babies don't have the ability to digest so they should avoid, watch for lactate intolerance for older children. Used in meat, poultry, biscuits, cheese, confectionary, wide ranges of foods. May be suitable for people lactose intolerant. Listed for UK, EU, USA, NZ, AU and CAN.
E326 **Potassium Lactate.** (Miscellaneous - Salts of Lactic Acid). Preservative,	$C_3H_5KO_3$ It is the potassium salt of lactic acid, see E270. Made from the bacterial fermentation of carbohydrates and molasses. Used in many foods including, ice cream, sweets, jam, cakes, meat and poultry products. Should not be given to babies and small children, as they have not yet

Acidity regulator.	developed the appropriate enzymes in the liver to metabolize these forms of lactate, watch for lactate intolerance for children. No known bad effects for adults in sources. See E325. Listed for UK, NZ, AU, USA, EU and CAN.
E327 **Calcium Lactate.** (Miscellaneou s - Salts of Lactic Acid). Preservative, Acidity regulator.	$C_6H_{10}CaO_6$ It is the calcium salt of lactic acid, see E270. Also see E326, E325. Made from the bacterial fermentation of carbohydrates and molasses. All fermented foods are naturally very rich in lactic acid. Used as an antacid, and to treat calcium deficiency, and as a baking powder. Also used in sweets, salad dressings, cakes, biscuits, meat, poultry, beer, yoghurt, soft drinks, canned fruit and vegetables. Should not be given to babies and small children, as they have not yet developed the appropriate enzymes in the liver to metabolize these forms of lactate, watch for lactate intolerance for older children. No known bad effects for adults in listed sources. Listed for UK, NZ, AU, EU, USA and CAN.
E328 **Ammonium lactate.** (Miscellaneou	$C_3H_9O_3N$ It is the ammonium salt of lactic acid. See E270, E325. It is made from the bacterial fermentation of milk. It is in sweets, salad dressings, cakes,

s - Salts of Lactic Acid Preservative). Acidity regulator.	biscuits, meat, poultry, beer, yoghurt, soft drinks, canned fruit, vegetables, wine, baked products and others. Small children should avoid, no known bad effects for adults. Can be in some lotions and may make skin more prone to sunburn. Excess ammonia is toxic, but it is naturally in the body as it is a product of protein catabolism and is safely removed by the by the liver. Normal blood ammonia levels range from 10-40 µmol/L. This increases 10% with exposure to 25 ppm, but is not considered harmful. People with liver dysfunction may be at increased risk for ammonia toxicity. Early symptoms of ammonia toxicity related to decreasing liver function include inability to concentrate, sleepiness and being prone to irritability. Avoid excess ingestion from manmade products. Not listed for EU, UK, USA and CAN. Listed for NZ and AU.
E329 **Magnesium lactate.** (Miscellaneou s - Salts of Lactic Acid).	$C_6H_{10}MgO_6$ It is the magnesium salt of lactic acid. See E270, E325. It is made from the bacterial fermentation of milk. In sweets, salad dressings, cakes, biscuits, meat and poultry, beer, yogurt, soft drinks, canned fruit and vegetables, wine, baked products,

Preservative, Acidity regulator.	jam, cheeses and others. Used as a mineral supplement to treat magnesium deficiency. It is also used to treat heartburn, indigestion, or stomach upset. Small children should avoid; no known bad effects for adults. Not listed for UK, USA, EU and CAN. Listed for NZ and AU.
E330 **Citric Acid.** (Miscellaneous - Citric Acid and its Salts). Preservative and acidifier.	$C_6H_8O_7$ It is naturally found in citrus fruits, such as oranges, lemons etc. It is a weak organic acid, a natural preservative and is used to add an acidic or sour taste to foods and soft drinks. It is made by the fermentation of carbohydrate solutions. Used in fruit juices, sauces, beers, baked goods, alcoholic drinks, cheese, spreads, cider, biscuits, cake mixes, frozen fish, ice-cream, jams, sweets, canned fruits, vegetables, and wine. It may cause intestine upset if in a concentrated amount, such as in some beverages. It damages tooth enamel in a strong concentration. Most citric acid is produced from corn (may be from GMO corn), manufacturers do not always take out the protein which may be hydrolyzed and create MSG (See E621) causing neurotoxin reactions in MSG-sensitive people. Be cautious of excess citric acid before strenuous

	exercise because it can cause stomach discomfort, heartburn and burping etc. In 2007 more than 50% of world's production is from China. Listed for UK, NZ, AU, EU, USA and CAN.
E331 **Sodium Citrates** **1. Monosodium citrate** **2. Disodium citrate** **3. Trisodium citrate.** (Miscellaneous - Citric Acid and its Salts). Sequestrant (binding agent), Anti-oxidant, Acidity regulator.	$C6H5Na3O7$ It is the sodium salt of citric acid, see E330. Made by the fermentation of carbohydrate solutions which may be corn based and may be GMO corn. It is a preservative and acid regulator. Used in gelatin products, jam, sweets, ice cream, milk powder, wine, carbonated beverages and cheeses. Can be found in popular energy drinks. Used as flavoring to give a tart taste. No known bad effects noted in sources. Listed for UK, EU, NZ, AU, USA and CAN.
E332 **Potassium Citrates** **1.Monopota**	$C_6H_5K_3O_7$ It is the potassium salt of citric acid, a weak acid found naturally in fruits. See E331. Made by the fermentation of carbohydrate solutions which may

ssium citrate **2.Tripotassium citrate.** (Miscellaneous - Citric Acid and its Salts). Acidity regulator.	be corn based and the corn may be genetically modified. Used in soft drinks, jams, sweets, ice-cream, carbonated beverages, wine, and cheese. It is a diuretic, can be used to treat gout and kidney stones. No known bad effects noted in sources. Listed for UK, NZ, AU, EU, USA and CAN.
E333 **Calcium Citrates** **1.Monocalcium citrate** **2.Dicalcium citrate** **3.Tricalcium citrate.** (Miscellaneous - Citric Acid and its Salts). Acidity regulator, Preservative, Anti-oxidant, Sequestrant (binding agent), Firming agent.	$Ca_3(C_6H_5O_7)_2$ It is the calcium salt of citric acid, a natural weak acid found in many fruits (has a sour taste). Made by the fermentation of carbohydrate solutions which may be corn based and the corn may be genetically modified. Used as firming agent in food. Used in gelatin products, ice cream, wine, carbonated beverages, sweets, jams, evaporated and condensed milk, milk powder, and processed cheeses etc. Used as a water softener because the citrate ions can chelate unwanted metal ions. It is used in some calcium supplements. See E331. No known bad effects noted in sources when used correctly in small amounts. Listed for UK, AU, NZ, USA, EU and CAN.

E334 **Tartaric Acid.** (Miscellaneous - Tartaric Acid and its Salts). Acidy regulator, Flavor enhancer, Stabilizer, Preservative.	$C_4H_6O_6$ It is naturally in fruit and wine, industrially synthesized as a by-product during wine making. An antioxidant used as an acidity regulator to give a sour taste and acts as a preservative in wine. Commonly combined with baking soda to be used as a leavening agent(Foaming action which lightens and softens breads or cakes etc). Used in chewing gum, jams, sweets, jelly, canned fruit and vegetables, baking powder, cocoa powder, and frozen dairy etc. No adverse effects noted in sources, when used moderately. Otherwise may cause stomach upset. Listed for UK, NZ, AU, EU, USA and CAN.
E335 **Sodium Tartrate 1.Monosodium tartrate 2.Disodium tartrate.** (Miscellaneous - Tartaric Acid and its Salts). Acidity regulator,	$C_4H_4Na_2O_6$ Or(2) $C_4H_8Na_2O_8$ It is a sodium salt of tartaric acid, see E334. Antioxidant and acidity regulator made as a by-product of the wine industry. Used in sweets, jelly, jams and carbonated beverages etc. No known bad effects when used moderately for most people. People with cardiac failure, high blood pressure, damaged liver or kidneys, and fluid retention need caution. Listed for AU, UK NZ, EU, USA and CAN.

Anti-Oxidant.	
E336 **Potassium Tartrate (Cream of Tartar)** **1.Monopotassium tartrate** **2.Dipotassium tartrate** (Miscellaneous - Tartaric Acid and its Salts). Acidity regulator, Anti-Oxidant.	$K_2C_4H_4O_6$ It is the potassium salt of tartaric acid, it is made as a by-product of the wine industry, see E334. Used in wine, citrus desserts, sweets, jelly, jams and soda drinks. There are no known bad effects if used moderately for most people. Those with kidney problems should use caution. Listed for NZ, UK, AU, EU, USA and CAN.
E337 **Potassium Sodium Tartrate Commonly knows as Seignette's salt or Rochelle salt.** (Miscellaneous – Tartaric	$KnaC_4H_4O_6 \cdot 4H_2O$ It is the potassium and sodium salt of tartaric acid, it is a double salt. Made as a by-product of the wine industry. Used in meat and cheese products, jams, and margarine. No known bad effects if used moderately for most people. People with kidney impairment should avoid, also those with heart problems or high blood pressure. See E335. Listed for UK, AU, NZ, CAN, USA and EU.

Acid and its Salts). Acidity regulator, Anti-Oxidant, Sequestrant (binding agent).	
E338 **Phosphoric acid** **or** **Orthophosphoric Acid.** (Miscellaneous - Phosphoric Acid and its Salts). Acidity regulator, Anti-Oxidant, Flavor enhancer.	H_3PO_4 It is a natural mineral inorganic acid that is mined primarily in the USA. It is a antioxidant and acidity regulator used inside carbonated beverages, processed meat, chocolate, fats and oils, beer, jam and sweets etc. Kidneys remove it by binding with calcium coming out of the bones and the whole body. If this is excessive over time it will lead to calcium deficiency and weak brittle bones, a caution for high soda drinkers. Excessive phosphate consumption can upset the internal mineral balance, and may cause kidney damage, osteoporosis (due to lack of adequate calcium in body, one possible cause of osteoporosis). Indicated as safe in listed sources with light ingestion, but avoid excessive ingestion. No more than 70 mg/kg of phosphoric acid per day, the less the better. Listed for USA,

	UK, AU, NZ, EU and CAN.
E339 **Sodium Phosphates 1.Monosodium phosphate 2.Disodium phosphate 3.Trisodium phosphate** **Other names, Sodium biphosphate or Sodium dihydrogen phosphate or Disodium hydrogen phosphate or Disodium orthophosphate or Sodium hydrogen phosphate or Disodium monohydrogen phosphate**	NaH_2PO_4 Or(2) Na_2HPO_4 Or(3) Na_3PO_4 It is the sodium salt of phosphoric acid, the phosphate being mined out of the ground. Used in cheeses, processed meats, powdered milk, coffee whiteners, cheese, jelly and baked foods etc. Excessive phosphate consumption may upset mineral balance in the body, it may cause kidney damage, and osteoporosis (due to lack of adequate calcium in body, one possible cause of osteoporosis). Indicated as safe in listed sources with light to very moderate ingestion. See E338. Listed for UK, AU, NZ, EU, USA and CAN.

or Phosphoric acid disodium salt. (Miscellaneous - Phosphoric Acid and its Salts). Acidity regulator, Buffer, Antioxidant, Emulsifier (mixing agent), Flavor enhancer.	
E340 **Potassium Phosphates** **1.Monopotassium phosphate** **2.Dipotassium phosphate** **3.Tripotassium phosphate**	KH_2PO_4 Or(2) K_2HPO_4 Or(3) K_3PO_4 It is the potassium salt of phosphoric acid, the phosphate mined out of the ground. Found in sauces, jelly products dessert mixes, meats, milk powders and hot chocolate mixes. Excessive phosphate consumption may upset the mineral balance inside the body, it also may cause kidney damage, and osteoporosis (due to lack of adequate calcium in body, one possible cause of osteoporosis). Indicated as safe in listed sources

Other names: dipotassium hydrogen phosphate, dipotassium hydrogen orthophosp hate, phosphoric acid dipotassium salt, potassium hydrogen phosphate. (Miscellaneou s - Phosphoric Acid and its Salts). Acidity regulator, Buffer, Antioxidant, Emulsifier (mixing agent).	with light to moderate ingestion. See E338. Listed for UK, AU, NZ, EU, USA and CAN.
E341 **Calcium Phosphates 1.Monocalci**	$Ca(H_2PO_4)_2$ Or(2) $CaHPO_4$ Or(3) $Ca_3(PO_4)_2$ It is the calcium salt of phosphoric acid, the phosphate is mined out of the ground. Used in self-raising flour,

um phosphate 2.Dicalcium phosphate 3.Tricalcium phosphate	baking powder, cake and mixes, in pre made cakes, other pastry products and in antacids. Used as antioxidant in food, an abrasive compound in toothpaste, as a firming agent, and in canned and packaged fruit deserts.
Other names, Phosphate, monobasic or monohydrate or Calcium tetrahydrogen diorthophosphate or Calcium hydrogen orthophosphate or Calcium phosphate dibasic or Tricalcium diorthophosphate or Calcium phosphate tribasic. (Miscellaneou	3. Synthetic tricalcium phosphate is added to table salt, sugar, baking powder and fertilizers to give a 'free-flowing' quality. Used in salt, sugar and other granular foods mixes, meats, milk powders, hot chocolate mixes.. See E338. Listed for UK, NZ, AU, USA, EU and CAN.

s - Phosphoric Acid and its Salts). Acidity regulator, Antioxidant, Anti-caking agent, Flour treatment agent.	
E342 **Ammonium phosphates** (Miscellaneous - Phosphoric Acid and its Salts). Acidity regulator, Firming agent, Leavening agent.	$H_9N_2O_4P$ It is the ammonium salt of phosphoric acid, the phosphate is mined out of the ground. Used in baked foods, alcoholic beverages, condiments, puddings, baking powder and margarine etc. Excessive ammonia may cause kidney and liver problems, not much information about Ammonium Phosphates. Excess ammonia is toxic, but naturally found in the body as it is a product of protein catabolism and is safely removed by the liver. Normal blood ammonia levels range from 10-40 µmol/L. This increases 10% with exposure to 25 ppm, but this level is not considered harmful. People with liver dysfunction can be at risk for ammonia toxicity. Early symptoms of ammonia toxicity related to decreasing liver function include

	inability to concentrate, sleepiness, and being prone to irritability. Not listed for EU and UK. Listed for AU, NZ, CAN and USA.
E343 **Magnesium phosphates** **1.Monomag nesium phosphate** **2.Dimagnesi um phosphate (Miscellane ous - Phosphoric Acid and its Salts)** Anti-oxidants, Anti-caking agents, Acidity regulators.	$Mg(H_2PO_4)_2$ Or(2) $MgHPO_4$ Or(3) $Mg_3(PO_4)_2$ It is the magnesium salt of phosphoric acid. The phosphate is mined out of the ground. An essential mineral, it is a non clumping agent found in salt substitutes. No adverse reactions noted in sources. See E338. Listed for UK, AU, NZ, EU, USA and CAN.
E344 **Lecithin citrate.** Acidity regulator, Preservative.	Not commonly used and not much information. Not listed for EU UK, USA, AU and NZ. Listed for CAN.

E345	$C_6H_6MgO_7$
Magnesium citrate. (Citric Acid Salt). Acidity regulator, Buffering agent. Vitamin mineral supplement.	It is the magnesium salt of citric acid, a natural weak acid found in fruits. Made commercially by the fermentation of carbohydrate solutions which may be made of corn or genetically modified corn or other GM plants or non modified plants. Used medicinally as a saline laxative and to completely empty the bowel prior to a major surgery or colonoscopy. It is available without a prescription and can be used as a magnesium supplement. It is also used for treatment of migraine headaches, but be careful not to overdose. Excreted by kidneys if overdosed, so those with kidney or liver problems be cautious. Appears safe in proper usage, caution about any excessive single vitamin or mineral supplementation for a long time as it may throw the body's mineral balance out of equilibrium. In general, clean food based vitamins are best for long term usage (years to decades), these should be more gentle on organs. Not listed for UK, AU, NZ, EU and USA. Allowed in CAN.
E349 **Ammonium**	$C_4H_8O_5N$ It is the ammonium salt of malic acid, a natural weak acid found in

malate (Malic Acid Salts). Acidity regulator, Buffer, Flavoring agent.	fruits. It gives food a tart taste. Used in beer, fruit juice concentrates, canned goods, frozen vegetables, soups, broths, ciders, vinegars, condiments, vegetables, sauces, batters, processed meats, breakfast cereals and snack foods. Considered unsuitable for infants and young children, may be related to skin irritations. Not much information. Excess ammonia is toxic, but found naturally inside the body as it is a product of protein catabolism and is safely removed by the by the liver. Normal blood ammonia levels range from 10-40 μmol/L. This increases 10% with exposure to 25 ppm, but this level is not considered harmful. People with liver dysfunction may be at increased risk for ammonia toxicity. Early symptoms of ammonia toxicity related to decreasing liver function include inability to concentrate, sleepiness and being prone to irritability. Not listed for UK, USA, EU and CAN. Listed for AU and NZ.
E350 **Sodium Malate or Sodium**	$C_4H_4Na_2O_5$ It is the sodium salt of Malic Acid. A low salt substitute, also used in fruit drinks and soft drinks. Malic acid, may be made from corn which in may be genetically modified. No

Hydrogen Malate. (Malic Acid Salts). Acidity regulator, Buffer, Flavoring agent	known adverse affects. Not listed for USA. Listed for UK, AU, NZ and EU.
E351 **Potassium malate.** (Malic Acid Salts). Acidity regulator, Buffer, Flavoring agent.	$C_4H_4K_2O_5$ It is the potassium salt of malic acid, a natural weak acid found in many fruits, commercially it is synthetically produced. May be used in canned vegetables, soups, sauces, fruit products, soft drinks, ice cream and fried foods etc. No adverse affects recorded in sources. See E350. Listed for UK, AU, NZ and EU. Not listed for CAN and USA.
E352 **Calcium malate.** (Malic Acid Salts). Acidity regulator, Buffer, Flavoring	$C_4H_4CaO_5$ It is the calcium salt of malic acid, a natural weak acid found in many fruits, commercially it is synthetically produced. May be used in canned vegetables, soups, sauces, fruit products, soft drinks, ice cream and fried foods etc. Used as a supplement. No adverse affects recorded in sources. See E350. Listed for UK, AU, NZ and EU. Not listed

agent.	for CAN and USA.
E353 **Metatartaric acid.** Acid. Preservative, Acid regulator.	$C8H8O10$ Metatartaric acid is made from tartaric acid, a natural organic acid that comes from the making of wine in the wine industry. Metatartaric acid is used to slow down or stop sedimentation in bottled wine. No known adverse reactions noted in sources. Listed for UK, AU, NZ and EU. Not listed for CAN and USA.
E354 **Calcium tartrate.** (Tartaric Salt). Preservative, Acid regulator.	$CaC_4H_4O_6$ It is the calcium salt of tartaric acid, a byproduct of the wine industry, prepared from wine fermentation dregs. It is a food acid and modifying agent in infant foods. No known bad effects noted in sources. Listed for UK, AU, NZ, EU and CAN. Not listed for USA.
E355 **Adipic acid** Acid, Acidity regulator, Buffer, Sequestrant (binding agent),	$C_6H_{10}O_4$ It is used in some calcium carbonate antacids to make them tart in flavor. Used in foods mostly as a gelling aid and for tartness. It's a synthetic food acid, only a small amount can be metabolized by humans and is listed as having mutating properties, and an eye irritant. It is a firming and raising agent when used in baking powder. Used in beer, fruit drinks, jams, pudding mixes, ice blocks and

Gelling agent, Leavening agent.	margarine etc. Toxic effects are found in rat studies including death, caution, limit or avoid it. Listed for UK, EU, NZ, AU, USA and CAN.
E356 **Sodium adipate.** (Salt of Acid). Acidy regulator. Anti oxidant.	$Na_2C_6H_8O_4$ The sodium salt of adipic acid, a natural acid present in beets and sugar cane, commercially it is synthetically made. It is an acidity regulator. It is used in herbal salts. Acceptable Daily Intake: Up to 5 mg/kg of body weight. No side effects noted in sources. It is metabolized in the body or excreted in the urine, considered safe in low amounts. See E355. Listed for UK and EU. Not listed for CAN, AU, NZ and USA.
E357 **Potassium adipate.** (Salt of Acid). Acidy regulator, Anti oxidant.	$K_2C_6H_8O_4$ The potassium salt of adipic acid, a natural acid present in beets and sugar cane, commercially it is synthetically made. It is a firming and raising agent in baked goods, beer, chewing gum, drinks, and desserts. No known bad effects noted in sources. See E355. Listed for AU, NZ, UK and EU. Not listed for CAN and USA.
E359 **Ammonium adipate.** (Salt of Acid).	$C_6H_{16}O_4N_2$ The ammonium salt of adipic acid a natural acid present in beets and sugar cane, commercially it is synthetically made. Indicated as

Acidy regulator. Anti oxidant.	somewhat new in sources. No known common uses, not much information. Excess ammonia is toxic, but it is naturally found in the body as it is a product of protein catabolism and is safely removed by the liver. Normal blood ammonia levels range from 10-40 µmol/L. This increases 10% with exposure to 25 ppm, but is not considered harmful. People with liver dysfunction may be at increased risk for ammonia toxicity. Early symptoms of ammonia toxicity related to decreasing liver function include inability to concentrate, sleepiness and being prone to irritability. Not listed for UK, EU, USA and CAN. Listed for AU and NZ.
E363 **Succinic acid.** Acid, Acidity regulator, Preservative, Flavor enhancer.	$C_4H_6O_4$ A natural acid found in most fruits and vegetables, commercially it is synthetically made. Global production is estimated at 16,000 to 30,000 tons a year, with an annual growth rate of 10%. Used in foods as a sequestrant (to remove impurities), buffer acidity regulator, preservative, flavor enhancer, and a neutralizing agent. Used in bakery items, breads, jellies, gelatin desserts and cake flavorings, pie fillings, cake mixes, dry mixes, baked goods, dairy,

	pickles, condiments, vinegar , sauces and oils etc. It may have an laxative effect and cause stomach intestinal problems. It needs more research as it is relativity new, caution. Some internet sources indicate it as safe, others not. Not listed for CAN and others. Listed for UK, AU, NZ, EU and USA.
E365 **Sodium fumarate.** (Salt of Acid). Acidity regulator, Anti-oxidant, Flavor enhancer, Raising agent.	$C_4H_2Na_2O_4$ It is the sodium salt of fumaric acid, that is naturally found in plants. Commercially, fumaric acid can be made by the catalytic oxidation of benzene, or by the fermentation of glucose. It may be made from corn which may be GMO corn. Used in baked foods, breads, fruit juices, wine, jams, gelatin, pie fillings, cake mixes, soft drinks, dry mixes, baking powder, dairy products, oils and fats, meat, eggs and nuts. May be used in dried, liquid, or frozen egg whites and artificial whipped cream etc. It strengthens bread dough, gives it an even grain and greater volume. No known bad effects noted in sources. Not listed for UK and EU. Listed for AU, NZ, CAN and USA.
E366 **Potassium fumarate.**	$K_2C_4H_2O_4$ The potassium salt of fumaric acid is naturally found in plants. Commercially fumaric acid can be

(Salt of Acid). Acidity regulator, Anti-oxidant, Flavor enhancer, Raising agent.	made by the catalytic oxidation of benzene, or by the fermentation of glucose. It may be made from corn and GMO corn. It acts as an acidity regulator, anti-oxidant, flavor enhancer, and a raising agent in flour based baked goods, and in processed foods. It regulates acidity in jams and makes gelatin set. Used in baked foods, breads, fruit juice, wine, jams, gelatin, pie fillings, cake mixes, soft drinks, dry mixes, baking powder, dairy products, oils and fats, meat, eggs and nuts. Used in dried, liquid or frozen egg whites and artificial whipped cream etc. No known bad effects noted in sources. Not listed for UK and EU. Listed for NZ, AU, CAN and USA.
E367 **Calcium fumarate.** (Salt of Acid). Acidity regulator, Anti-oxidant, Flavor enhancer, Raising agent	$CaC_4H_2O_4$ The calcium salt of formaric acid is naturally found in plants. Commercially fumaric acid can be made by the catalytic oxidation of benzene, or by the fermentation of glucose. It may be made from corn and GMO corn. It is an acidity regulator, and used to fortify foods and beverages with calcium, to improve the texture in fruits and vegetables. It is used in breads, fruit juice, wine, dry mixes, jellies, jams, gelatin, pie fillings, cake mixes, soft

	drinks, baking powder, baked goods and dairy products, etc. No known bad effects noted in sources. Not listed for EU and UK. Listed for NZ, AU, CAN and USA.
E368 **Ammonium fumarate.** (Salt of Acid). Acidity regulator, Flavor enhancer.	$C_4H_{10}N_2O_4$ The ammonium salt of fumaric acid is naturally found in plants. Commercially fumaric acid can be made by the catalytic oxidation of benzene, or by the fermentation of glucose. It may be made from corn and GMO corn. Fairly new, not much information. Excess ammonia is toxic, but found naturally in the body as it is a product of protein catabolism and is safely removed by the by the liver. Normal blood ammonia levels range from 10-40 µmol/L. This increases 10% with exposure to 25 ppm, but is not considered harmful. People with liver dysfunction may be at increased risk for ammonia toxicity. Early symptoms of ammonia toxicity related to decreasing liver function include inability to concentrate, sleepiness and being prone to irritability. Not listed for UK, EU, USA and CAN. Listed for AU and NZ.
E370 **1,4-**	It is commercially synthesized from hydroxycarboxylic acid. It is used as an acid regulator, for artificial

Heptonolact one. Acid Regulator. Sequestrant (binding agent).	flavoring, and as a sequestrant (to remove impurities). Used in dried soups, powdered desserts and to make artificial flavors-coconut, nut, and vanilla. Not listed for UK, NZ, USA, CAN, AU, EU and some other countries.
E375 **Niacin or Nicotinic acid or Nicotinamid e.** Color Retention, Anti oxidant.	$C_6NH_5O_2$ It is a B vitamin, used in food as a color retention agent as well as a B3 vitamin. Commercially it is made from nicotine It is essential for health. Typical products include bread, flour, and cereal. As a supplement very helpful for people with clogged arteries, it causes a hot flashe when taken-a short term artificially created fever with hot skin and flushing. At doses in excess of 1,000-2,000 mg per day may cause liver damage, diabetes, gastritis, eye damage, and elevated blood levels of uric acid (which may cause gout); at amounts as low as 50-100 mg may cause red skin flushing (harmless but somewhat painful), headache, and stomach-ache if taken on an empty stomach. Be cautious of the slow release form of Niacin supplements and any other modified forms of Niacin, you may want to stick with the regular kinds of Niacin, consult

	with your health care provider. No known bad effects when normally used as a food additive. Not listed for UK, NZ, AU and CAN. Listed for USA.
E380 **Triammoni um citrate** (Salt of Acid). Acidity regulator, Buffer, Emulsifier (mixing agent).	$C6H8O7.3H3N$ The ammonium salt of citric acid, a natural weak acid found fruit. Commercially it can be made by the fermentation of carbohydrate solutions, usually molasses or hydrolyzed corn starch; source carbohydrate may or may not be genetically modified (GMO corn etc). Used in chocolate, confectionary, and cheese spreads. It may interfere with liver and pancreas function - more study needed, caution. Listed for UK, NZ, AU and EU. Not listed for USA and CAN.
E381 **Ammonium ferric citrates.** (Salt of Acid). Anti caking agent, Supplement.	$C_6H_{5+4y}Fe_xN_yO_7$ It is a mixture of ammonia, iron, and citric acid-a natural acid found in fruit. Commercially it may be produced by the fermentation of carbohydrate solutions; usually molasses or hydrolyzed corn starch the source carbohydrate may or may not be genetically modified (GMO corn), it also can be made from citric acid. Used as an anti-caking agent in salt, and to enrich the iron content of food. Used in sodas, salt, and as a

	source of iron in iron-fortified breakfast foods, cereals and infant formulas. Can be unsafe in high dosages. No known bad effects in normal food additive usage. Excess ammonia is toxic, but naturally in the body as it is a product of protein catabolism and is safely removed by the by the liver. Normal blood ammonia levels range from 10-40 µmol/L. This increases 10% with exposure to 25 ppm, but is not considered harmful. People with liver dysfunction may be at increased risk for ammonia toxicity. Early symptoms of ammonia toxicity related to decreasing liver function include inability to concentrate, sleepiness and being prone to irritability. Not listed for UK, EU and CAN. Listed for AU, NZ and USA.
E383 **Calcium glycerylphosphate or Calcium glycerophosphate.** Acidy regulator Supplement.	$C_3H_7CaO_6P$ Used to fortify foods and as a supplement in baked foods and dairy products etc. Appears to be safe, but not much information, caution. Have caution of using any single vitamin or mineral over a long period of time (months to years and decades) at high dosages because it may throw the body out of balance. Caution when taking any non food based supplement long term as it may

	strain the organs when processing it. Not listed for NZ, AU and EU. Listed for USA and CAN.
E384 **Isopropyl citrate.** Acidity regulator Sequestrant, (binding agent), Anti oxidant.	$C_9H_{14}O_7$ Made by esterifying citric acid with 2-propanol, it is a combination of citric acid and isopropyl alcohol. It may interfere with results of medical lab tests if inside body during testing. Used in oils and fats, fat spreads. Not much information. Not listed for UK, EU, NZ, AU and CAN. Listed for USA.
E385 **Calcium Disodium EDTA or EDTA.** Emulsifiers and Stabilizers.	$C_{10}H_{16}N_2O_8$ It is the calcium salt of disodium ethylene diamine tetraacetate. It is a colorless, water-soluble material used as a chelating agent, emulsifying salt, anti-oxidant, preservative, stabilizer, and as a sequestrant. It is a synthetic flavor, a texture retainer, an anti-gushing agent in beer, a preservative and color promoter. Causes mineral imbalances, a enzyme and blood coagulant inhibitor. It may cause gastrointestinal disturbances, blood in urine, kidney damage and muscle cramps. It may cause errors in medical lab tests if inside the body from food additives. Used in sodas, salad dressings, egg products, potato

	salad, lima beans, mushrooms and sandwich spreads. Used in lard, canned legumes, creamed turkey, fats and oils, potatoes and french fries, dried bananas, fruit juices, canned seafood, cereal, ham, bacon, hotdogs, milk, canned vegetables, egg custards, mayonnaise, salad dressings, canned apples, cheese, frozen ground beef, processed vegetables and fruit etc. Not listed for AU. Listed for UK, AU, NZ, USA, EU and CAN.
E387 **Oxystearin.** Antioxidant, Sequestrant(b inding agent).	It is a mixture of glycerides of stearic acid and other fatty acids. A metal scavenger and stabilizer used to prevent crystallization in fats and oils. Used in oils and fats, sugar, yeast products etc. Acceptable Daily Intake: Up to 25 mg/kg of body weight. Used in vegetable oils and fats, canola oil, sunflower seed oil, sesame seed oil, soybean oils, maize oil, safflower oil, cottonseed oil, rapeseed oil, mustard seed oil, and margarine, beet sugar, and yeast. No known acute side effects in commonly used concentrations. The body treats it as fat. Caution, it may build up toxins over time in stored body fat.
E388	It is a synthetic compound an anti-oxidant. Used in fats, oils, and drinks

Thiodipropi onic acid. Antioxidant.	that are prone to oxidation, used mainly in cosmetics. Acceptable Daily Intake: Up to 3 mg/kg body weight. No known side effects in commonly used concentrations. May build up toxins in the body fat over time with continuous usage.
E392 **Extracts of Rosemary.** Medicinal Herb, Flavoring agent.	Rosemary is a woody, perennial herb with fragrant, evergreen, needle-like leaves and white, pink, purple or blue flowers. It is part of the mint family. The leaves have a bitter astringent taste, highly aromatic, and are used in many foods for flavor in home cooking. Folklore indicates it improves memory. Rosemary in culinary or therapeutic doses is generally safe, but can cause allergic skin reactions when used in topical preparations. According to recent European research, rosemary interferes with the absorption of iron and shouldn't be consumed by people with iron deficiency. Extremely rare, but it can cause epileptic seizures in sensitive people. Avoid ingesting large amounts especially if pregnant or breast feeding. No information about commercial usage as a food additive. Allowed in EU in 2010, may see increasing usage. Not listed for UK, AU, NZ and CAN. Listed for USA.

Emulsifiers & Stabilizers E400-E495:

Emulsifiers allow water and oils to remain mixed together in an emulsion, examples are mayonnaise, ice cream, and homogenized milk.

Stabilizers, thickeners and gelling agents, like agar or pectin (used in jam for example) give foods a firmer texture. While they are not true emulsifiers, they help to stabilize mixtures of foods, to prevent them from separating into layers.

Natural gums are capable of causing a large viscosity increase in a solution, even with using small concentrations. In the food industry they are used as thickening agents, gelling agents, emulsifying agents, and stabilizers. In other industries, they are also used as adhesives, binding agents, clarifying agents, encapsulating agents, swelling agents and foam stabilizers, etc. In nature most often these gums are found in the woody elements of plants or in seed coatings.

| E400

Alginic Acid.

(Emulsifiers and Stabilizers - other plant gums).
Emulsifier(mixing agent), | $(C_6H_8O_6)_n$
Alginic Acid is extracted from the cell walls of brown algae, it is a flavorless gum that is put into food to increase viscosity, and to be a emulsifier, thickener, and stabilizer. It is absorbed by water, which makes it very useful in dehydrated products. Alginic acid, (alginato) is also used in culinary arts, most notably, where natural juices of fruits and vegetables are encapsulated in bubbles that |

Thickener, Stabilizer.	explode on the tongue when consumed. Due to its ability to absorb water quickly, alginate can be changed through a lyophilization process to a new structure that has the ability to expand. This is used in the weight loss industry as an appetite suppressant. In March, 2010 researchers at Newcastle University announced that dietary alginates can reduce human fat uptake by more than 75%. As a food additive it is used as a thickener and vegetable gum, made from seaweed As a artificial sweetener, it is used in custard mix, cordial, flavored milk, ice blocks, pastry, jelly, ice cream, cheese, confectionary, canned icing, beer thickened cream and yogurt. No known bad effects in small quantities for most people, large quantities may prevent absorption of some nutrients, so it may cause deficiency when used for a long time weight loss supplement. Some people may have adverse reactions, such as eye, skin and gastrointestinal problems. Pregnant women should avoid, people with heart, blood pressure or kidney problems may need to avoid. Some salts of Alginic Acid may be used as a low sodium salt

	replacement. The algae extract is called Carrageenan, see E407. Listed for UK, AU, NZ, EU, USA and CAN.
E401 **Sodium Alginate.** Emulsifiers and Stabilizers – other plant gums. Emulsifier(mixing agent), Thickener, Stabilizer.	$NaC_6H_7O_6$ It is the sodium salt of alginic acid, see E400. Listed for UK, AU, NZ, EU, USA and CAN.
E402 **Potassium Alginate.** (Emulsifiers and Stabilizers - other plant gums). Emulsifier(mixing agent), Thickener, Stabilizer.	$KC_6H_7O_6$. It is the potassium salt of Alginic Acid, see E400. Listed for UK, AU, NZ, EU, USA and CAN.
E403	$C_{13}H_{16}N_3NaO_4S$ It is the ammonium salt of Alginic

Ammonium Alginate. (Emulsifiers and Stabilizers - other plant gums). Emulsifier(mixing agent), Thickener, Stabilizer.	Acid, see E400. Excess ammonia is toxic, but found naturally in the body as a product of protein catabolism and is safely removed by the by the liver. Normal blood ammonia levels range from 10-40 µmol/L. This increases 10% with exposure to 25 ppm, but not considered harmful at this level. People with liver dysfunction may be at increased risk for ammonia toxicity. Early symptoms of ammonia toxicity related to decreasing liver function include inability to concentrate, sleepiness and being prone to irritability. Listed for UK, AU, NZ, EU, USA and CAN.
E404 **Calcium Alginate.** (Emulsifiers and Stabilizers – other plant gums). Emulsifier(mixing agent), Thickener, Stabilizer.	$(C_{12}H_{14}CaO_{12})_n$ It is the calcium salt of Alginic Acid, see E400. Listed for UK, AU, NZ, EU, USA and CAN.
E405	$(C9H14O7o)n$ Chemically propylene glycol alginate

Propylene glycol alginate or Propane-1,2-Diol Alginate (Emulsifiers and Stabilizers - other plant gums). Emulsifier(mixing agent), Thickener, Stabilizer.	is an ester of Alginic Acid, which is derived from kelp or from petroleum. Used as a artificial sweetener base, preservative, used in germicides, paint remover and antifreeze Used in custard mixes, yoghurt, jelly, ice-creams, flavored milk, artificial sweetener, salad dressings, canned icing, cheese, as well as being in weight lost supplements and indigestion or heart burn pills. It also inhibits the absorption of strontium, one of the more toxic components of nuclear fallout. Adverse reactions are noted as common enough for concern, avoid in pregnancy. Caution. Listed for UK, NZ, AU, EU, USA and CAN.
E406 **Agar.** (Emulsifiers and Stabilizers - other plant gums). Gelling agent, Thickener, Stabilizer.	$(C_{12}H_{18}O_9)n$ Agar-Agar is a gelatinous substance obtained from the cell walls of red seaweed. It is used in food as a natural gelling agent, because it is a seaweed gum. Not digestible, therefore it acts as source of dietary fiber. Typical products include ice cream, frozen desserts, icings, sweets, fondants, milk cream, milk, yogurt and can be used as a laxative. No known bad effects in normal usage, but may gum up the system if used in great excess. It is a common ingredient used for cooking, better

	than many other less healthy thickening and gelling agents. Listed for UK, AU, NZ, USA, EU and CAN.
E407 And E407(a) **Carrageenan, E407. and Processed euchuema seaweed, (407a).** E407(a) differs from E407 mainly because it has a lot of cellulose. (Emulsifiers and Stabilizers - other plant gums). Gelling agent, Thickener, Stabilizer.	Carrageenan is a fiber extracted from seaweed used as a thickener or stabilizer. There are different kinds of molecular structures for carrageenan, there are three main ones in use. 1. Kappa-carrageenan, it is used mostly in breading and batter due to its gelling nature. 2. Lambda carrageenan, is used as a non gelling variety, that assists in retaining moisture and in contributing to viscosity in sweet doughs. 3. Iota carrageenan, is used primarily in fruit applications. Degraded concentrated carrageenan, which is not a permitted additive, may cause major health problems such as cancer, ulcers and damage to the immune system. Degraded carrageenan is something that has degraded into a different form. The danger is if the degraded or non permitted form of carrageenan being used at a too great of concentration in the whole mass of carrageenan, the limit should be no more than 5% of total. Also it is possible to have chemical contaminated carrageenan. Pure natural carrageenan appears

	safe, but more study is needed, Used in many products such as soy milk, processed meats, beer, ice-cream, milk shakes, sweetened condensed milk, sauces and desserts. Carrageenan is a vegetarian and a vegan alternative to gelatin and some forms of carrageenan has a history of hundreds of years in usage. It is on the FDA list for more study, caution it has potential for adverse reactions, not for small children. In test animals carrageenan can cause intestinal troubles, ulcers and malignancies. See E400. Listed for UK, AU, NZ, EU, USA and CAN.
E408 **Furcellaran or Danish agar.** (Emulsifiers and Stabilizers - other plant gums). Gelling agent Thickener Stabilizer.	It is made from the seaweed Furcellaria Fastigiata as a gelatinous substance. The structure of furcellaran is similar to that of kappa carrageenan and can be described as a hybrid of the kappa/beta carrageenans complex. Used in soy milk and processed meats, beer, ice-cream, milk shakes, sweetened condensed milk, sauces and desserts etc. It may be used in diabetic products. Daily Intake: Up to 75 mg/kg body weight. No known bad effects in proper usage, but high concentrations may bring about flatulence and bloating, due to fermentation by the intestinal micro

	flora. Similar to E407, sometimes named E407. Not listed for UK, EU, AU, NZ and USA. Listed for CAN.
E409 **Aribinogala ctan** **or** **Larch Gum.** (Emulsifiers and Stabilizers - other plant gums). Thickener.	It is a natural polysaccharide extracted by water from Western larch wood. Used as a thickener and stabilizer in foods. It is in essential oils, sweeteners, pudding mixes, and flavor bases. A small percentage of people, less than 3%, may experience bloating and flatulence if given Larch Gum as a medicine, it has many possible uses as an inexpensive medicine. Bad reactions are possible for some people, more research is needed, caution. Mixed information from different sources saying it is good or bad. Not listed for UK, EU, USA and CAN. Listed for AU and NZ.
E410 **Locust Bean Gum** **or** **Carob Bean Gum.** (Emulsifiers and Stabilizers - other plant gums). Thickener,	Vegetable gum is extracted from the seeds of the Locust/Carob tree mostly found in the Mediterranean. It is used as a thickening and gelling agent in food. The bean, when made into powder, is sweet with a flavor similar to chocolate, it is used to sweeten foods and as a chocolate substitute (carob chocolate chips is the common product). Used in fruit juice drinks, dressings, ice-creams, and as a non caffeinated substitute for chocolate. May lower cholesterol, and is soluble in hot water. Safe in

Gelling agent.	small to moderate amounts for most people. Large amounts may cause abdominal pain, diarrhea, cough in infants and other adverse reactions. Gauge how you feel in it's use as a chocolate substitute. Listed for UK, AU, NZ, EU, USA and CAN.
E411 **Oat Gum** (Emulsifiers and Stabilizers - other plant gums). Stabilizer Thickener.	It is a natural polysaccharide, produced from oats. In high amounts it may cause flatulence and bloating, due to fermentation by the intestinal micro flora, the same for all indigestible polysaccharides. Considered safe enough, but hardly used in industry as an additive. Not listed for UK, EU, AU and NZ. Listed for USA and CAN.
E412 **Guar Gum** (Emulsifiers and Stabilizers - other plant gums). Emulsifier, (mixing agent), Thickener, Stabilizer.	It is primarily the ground endosperm of guar beans. The guar bean is mostly grown in India and Pakistan. The drought-resistant guar bean can be eaten as a green bean, fed to cattle or used in green manure. Unlike locust bean gum, it is not self-gelling. However, either borax or calcium can be cross-link guar gum, causing it to gel. It is eight times more thickening than cornstarch. It is sometimes fed to cattle in the US. It may cause nausea, flatulence and cramps. Used in bakeries, dairies, dressings, sauces, and in processed meats and

	may reduce cholesterol. Safe in proper usage for most people. Listed for UK, NZ, AU, EU, USA and CAN.
E413 **Tragacanth Gum.** (Emulsifiers and Stabilizers - other plant gums). Emulsifier (mixing agent), Thickener, Stabilizer.	It is a natural polysaccharide produced from the dried sap of middle eastern legumes of the genus *Astragalus*, Iran is the biggest producer of the best quality gum. The sap is a viscous, odorless, tasteless, water-soluble, mixture of polysaccharides that are drained from the tree, dried and then ground into powder. It is less common in products than other gums, such as gum arabic or guar gum, largely because most tragacanth is grown in middle eastern countries which have shaky trade relations with western countries where the gum is to be used. Commercial cultivation of tragacanth plants has generally not proved economically worthwhile in the West since cheaper gums can be used for similar purposes Used as an emulsifier, thickener, and stabilizer. It is in salad dressings, cream cheese, cottage cheese, cake icing, processed cheese, and, ice cream. Be cautious if you suffer from allergies or intolerances. It may cause asthma attacks, diarrhea, gas, constipation and skin rashes, a potential contact allergen. Listed for UK, AU, NZ, EU,

	USA and CAN.
E414 **Gum Acacia or Gum Arabic.** (Emulsifiers and Stabilizers - other plant gums). Thickener, Glazing agent, Emulsifier(mixing agent), Stabilizer.	It is a natural polysaccharide which is produced from the dried gum of the stems and branches of the Acacia tree. Grown in Sudan, Chad, and Nigeria, which in 2007 all together produced 95% of world exports. It is easily broken down by the human digestive system. Typical products include chewing gum, sweets, jelly, fondants, beer, soft drinks, fruit squash, and wine. It can be an irritant and has the potential for allergic reactions. It may cause asthma and skin rashes etc. Listed for UK, AU, NZ, EU, USA and CAN.
E415 **Xanthan Gum** (Emulsifiers and Stabilizers - other plant gums). Thickening agent, Stabilizer, Emulsifier (mixing	$C_{35}H_{49}O_{29}$ Xanthan gum may be derived from a variety of source products that are themselves common allergens, such as corn, wheat, dairy, or soy. People with known sensitivities or allergies to such food products are advised to avoid foods including generic xanthan gum or determine the source of the xanthan gum. Used in salad dressings and sauces etc. Extracted by chemical process, if poorly done it may leave toxins behind. Avoid if sensitive to gluten, adverse reactions include intestinal

agent).	bloating and diarrhea. Generally safe enough for most people but be careful with very small children and infants with allergies. Listed for UK, AU, NZ, EU, USA and CAN.
E416 **Karaya gum.** (Emulsifiers and Stabilizers - other plant gums). Thickening agent, Stabilizer, Emulsifier (mixing agent).	Karaya Gum is a polysaccharide made from the tree Sterculia Urens. It is used as a thickening agent, stabilizer, and emulsifier in foods. It can be used with E410 to increase the shelf-life of baked goods. It can multiply its volume by a hundred times with water, so it makes a good food filler agent. Used in fillings, sauces, cereals, cheese spreads desserts, nut coatings, dairy products, chewing gum and dietary food supplements. Can be used as a laxative. It has potential for adverse reactions, such as asthma, hives, skin rash, itchy skin, and stuffy/runny nose and gastrointestinal upsets. Listed for UK, NZ, AU, EU, USA and CAN.
E417 **Tara gum** (Emulsifiers and Stabilizers - other plant gums).	Tara is a small leguminous tree or thorny shrub native to Peru. Tara gum is a white or beige, nearly odorless powder that is produced by separating and grinding the endosperm of C. spinosa seeds. A solution of tara gum is less viscous than guar gum solution of the same concentration, but more viscous than

Thickening agent, Stabilizer, Emulsifier (mixing agent).	a solution of locust bean gum. Medicinal uses common in Peru include gargling infusions of the pods for inflamed tonsils or washing wounds; it is also used for fevers, colds and stomach aches. Water from boiled dried pods is also used to kill fleas and other insects. Used in ice cream, cosmetics and fast food preparations. There are no known bad effects inside foods listed in sources. Listed for NZ, UK, AU and EU. Not listed for CAN and USA.
E418 **Gellan gum.** (Emulsifiers and Stabilizers - other plant gums). Thickening agent, Stabilizer, Emulsifier (mixing agent).	Used primarily as a gelling agent, an alternative to agar in microbiological culture. It is able to withstand 120 °C heat, making it especially useful in culturing thermophilic organisms, soluble in water. One needs only approximately half the amount of gellan gum as agar to reach an equivalent gel strength. Used in Soy milks to keep the soy protein suspended in milk. It is used in juices, gel drinks, dressings, and dairy products, no known bad effects. Listed for UK, AU, NZ, USA, EU and CAN.
E419 **Ghatti gum or Indian gum.**	This gum is made from a small to medium-sized tree native to the India. The common English name for this gum is Axlewood. It is used in beverages, and butter. In 2007 high

(Emulsifiers and Stabilizers - other plant gums). Thickening agent, Stabilizer, Emulsifier (mixing agent).	amounts of dioxin were found in Ghatti gum shipments to EU. This prompted a strict regulation for Ghatti gum imports into the EU, but may not be in place for other countries. No information found for adverse reactions either way. Not listed for UK, NZ, AU, EU and CAN. Listed for USA.
E420 **Sorbitol.** (Sugar Alcohols). Sweetener, Humectant (retains moisture).	$C_6H_{14}O_6$ Artificial sweetener, derived from glucose, either obtained from berries of the Sorbus aucuparia tree or synthesized from glucose. Used as a tabletop sweetener and is inside many foods labeled "diet" as a sugar substitute. It has about 60% of the sweetness of sugar, with a sweet taste that gives a cooling sensation. It is often used in diet foods including diet drinks and ice cream, mints, cough syrups, and sugar-free chewing gum. Used in ice-cream, soft drinks, chewing gum, baked goods, chocolate, jams, canned fruits, frozen desserts, cookies, cakes, icings and fillings, marshmallows, preserves, jellies, vinegar, pickles, salad dressings, beer, tea, coffee, flavored drinks, toothpastes, mouthwashes

	and cosmetics. Can be used as a laxative, may be in dried fruits and may contribute to the laxative effect of prunes. Not suitable for diabetics, infants and young children, it may cause liver toxicity, gastrointestinal upsets and intestinal pain. Prohibited in foods for infants and young children. Sorbitol ingestion of 20 grams (0.7 oz) per day from sugar-free gum has led to severe diarrhea leading to unintended weight loss of 11 kilograms (24 lb) in eight months, for a woman originally weighing 52 kilograms (110 lb). (Source is Wikipedia) Not recommended for diabetics or people with fructose intolerance. Listed for UK, AU, NZ, EU, USA and CAN.
E421 **Mannitol or 1,2,3,4,5,6-hexanehexol, Mannite or Manna sugar.** (Sugar Alcohols) Sweetener,	$C_6H_{14}O_6$ Artificial sweetener and humectant (helps to keep food moist), extracted from seaweed or the manna ash tree, but mostly manufactured commercially from different kinds of sugars.. Typical products are low calorie sugar-free foods. Mannitol and sorbitol are isomers, which means same molecular formula, but different physical shape. Mannitol does not stimulate an increase in blood glucose, and is therefore used as a sweetener for people with

Humectant (retains moisture).	diabetes, and in chewing gums. It also has a low glycemic index, The pleasant taste and mouth feel of mannitol also makes it a popular for chewable tablets. Used in chewable tablets, chewing gum, baked goods, chocolates, sauces, frozen fish, and mustard. Not for infants and young children, or those with kidney and/or liver impairment. If used in excess it may cause bloating and diarrhea. Linked to hyperactivity, kidney damage. Listed for UK, AU, NZ, USA, EU and CAN.
E422 **Glycerol.** (Sugar Alcohols). Sweetener, Humectant (retains moisture), Thickening agent- (in liquids), Filler, Bulking agent.	$C_3H_8O_3$ Sweetener and humectant (helps to keep food moist), it is a oily, colorless liquid alcohol, made by decomposition of natural fats with alkalis. It is usually a by-product of soap making using animal fat or vegetable oil, or can be made from propylene or fermented from sugar. Currently the main source for Glycerol is as a byproduct of biodiesel. It is projected that by the year 2020 production will be six times more than demand because of mandated increases of bio diesel fuel, which may prompt a search for expanding the market for Glycerol. It is used in flexible coatings on sausages and cheeses, also in

	crystallized and dried fruit, liqueurs and vodka, cookies and biscuits, baked goods, ice-cream, dried fruit, soft drinks, marshmallows, toothpastes, low calorie foods and more. Large quantities can cause headaches, thirst, nausea, eye skin irritations and high blood sugar levels. Sensitive people may have adverse reaction with small amounts. Listed for UK, NZ, AU, EU, USA and CAN.
E424 **Curdlan Gum.** Firming agent, Gelling agent, Thickener, Stabilizer.	$(C_6H_{10}O_5)_n$ A natural polysaccharide that is produced commercially by the bacterial fermentation of the mutant strain of Alcaligenes faecalis. It is widely used by food processors in Taiwan to improve texture and crispness. It may be in fish or sea food paste which in turn is used in seafood cakes to cut cost. Processing companies usually do not add curdlan gum at an amount higher than 6 percent, since a content of 10 percent or more may harden the foodstuff, making it non chewable. Not much information about safety, available information indicates it is safe enough, except that too much may cause indigestion. Available information indicates that it is not used by western countries to date.

	Not listed for UK, AU, NZ, EU, USA and CAN.
E425 **Konjac, or Konjac gum or Konjac glucomanna ne.** Gelling agent, Emulsifier.	The plant Konjac is grown to make a flour or jelly. The jelly is a highly viscous solution that is almost tasteless, and is used as a gelling agent and emulsifier in foods. In candies it will not melt in the mouth (water will not help it dissolve) so can present a serious choking hazard especially with small children, it may also cause intestinal blockages. It is banned in Australia. It is popular as an Asian fruit jelly snack and other foods in Asian countries. In the United States it is commonly in lychee cups or konjac candy, usually served in bite-sized plastic cups. Listed for UK and EU. Not listed for AU, NZ, CAN and USA.
E426 **Soybean hemicellulo se.** Emulsifier (mixing agent), Stabilizer, Thickener, Gelling agent.	It is a cell wall polysaccharide that is extracted from soy fiber using dilute sodium hydroxide. Can be used in baked goods and low calorie breads, including muffins, cookies and crackers, frozen foods, yogurt drinks, anti caking agent in noodles and rice. Should avoid if allergic to soy, source soy may be genetically modified. Not much information either way on safety. Listed for UK and EU. Not listed for AU, NZ, CAN and USA. http://ec.europa.eu/food/fs/sc/scf/o

	ut187_en.pdf
E427 **Cassia gum.** Emulsifier (mixing agent), Stabilizer, Thickener. See E499 http://www.cassiagums.com/about_cassia_gums.html	E427 and E499 have the same name, 'Cassia gum' and the information I find indicates they are the same or very similar. See E499
E429 **Peptones.** Processing aid, Supplement.	Peptones are short polymers of amino acid monomers linked by peptide bonds. They are like proteins, but differ in the size as they are smaller. Peptones are derived from animal milk or meat digested by proteolytic digestion. In addition to containing small peptides, the resulting spray-dried material includes fats, metals, salts, vitamins and many other biological compounds. Peptone is used in nutrient media for growing bacteria and fungi in science and industry. Used as nutrient supplement for amino acids, vitamins, particularly B-complexes. Source protein may be

	pork. Caution may be partially hydrolyzed, therefore hard to digest for some people and may clog arteries and heart, the degree determined by the amount digested and genetics, it may contain MSG. Not listed for UK, AU, NZ, EU and CAN. Listed for USA.
E430 **Polyoxyethane (8) Stearate or Polyoxyl 8 stearate.** (Emulsifiers and Stabilizers - Fatty Acid derivatives). Emulsifier (mixing agent), Gelling agent, Stabilizer, Thickener.	It is a synthetic compound, produced from ethylene oxide (another synthetic compound) and stearic acid (a natural fatty acid). It is mainly used in sauces and cosmetics. Acceptable Daily Intake, up to 25 mg/kg of body weight. Usually no noticeable side effects in concentrations used for most people. People sensitive to propylene glycol should also avoid E430-E436. Potential to cause cancer, it needs more study. It may be best to avoid excessive regular usage. Not listed for UK, AU, NZ, EU and USA. Listed for CAN.
E431 **Polyoxyethane (40) Stearate**	It is a synthetic compound produced from a mixture of mono- and diesters of edible stearic acid, with polyoxyethylene diols. Acceptable daily intake is up to 25 mg/kg of

(Emulsifiers and Stabilizers - Fatty Acid derivatives). Emulsifier (mixing agent),	body weight. Primarily used in bakery products, and puddings, it may cause skin allergy in some people. Usually no adverse effects in concentrations used for most people. People sensitive to propylene glycol should avoid E430-E436. A possible cancer causing agent, relatively new in usage and needs more research. Listed for UK, NZ, AU and EU. Not listed for USA and CAN.
E432 **Polysorbate 20** **or** **Polyoxyethy lene sorbitan monolaurat e.** (Emulsifiers and Stabilizers - Fatty Acid derivatives). Emulsifier (mixing agent), Improve texture.	$C_{58}H_{114}O_{26}$ It is a synthetic compound, produced from ethylene oxide (also a synthetic compound) and stearic acid (a natural fatty acid). It is used with other emulsifiers to disperse flavors and colors, to improve texture in bakery goods, to make essential oils and vitamins soluble in water. Acceptable daily intake is up to 25 mg/kg of body weight. Used in ice-creams, soft drinks, and baked goods. No noticeable bad effects in the concentrations used for most people. People sensitive to propylene glycol should also avoid E430-E436. It is banned in Australia and some other countries, it may cause cancer and needs more research. Listed for UK, USA and EU. Not listed for CAN, AU and NZ. .
E433	$C_{64}H_{124}O_{26}$

Polysorbate 80, or Polyoxyethylene (20) sorbitan monooleate. (Emulsifiers and Stabilisers - Fatty Acid derivatives). Emulsifier (mixing agent).	A synthetic compound that is produced by the esterification of polyethoxylated sorbitan and oleic acid. Added to foods as an emulsifier, it is a viscous water-soluble yellow liquid. Acceptable daily intake is up to 25 mg/kg of body weight. Used in bakery products and ice cream. It is also used in some kinds of eye drops. It may increase the absorption of fat-soluble substances. No noticeable bad side effects in the concentrations used for most people. People sensitive to propylene glycol should avoid the group of E430-E436. It may be contaminated by 1,4 dioxane, a potential toxin. It may cause cancer, a possible allergen, and needs more study. Listed for UK, AU, NZ, EU, USA and CAN.
E434 **Polysorbate 40 or Polyoxyethane (20) Sorbitan Monopalmitate.** (Emulsifiers and Stabilisers -	$C_{22}H_{42}O_6.(C_2H_4O)n$ It is made from ethylene oxide, sorbitol and palmitic acid. Used in baked goods and cakes. Acceptable daily intake is up to 25 mg/kg of body weight. No noticeable bad effects in concentrations used for most people. People sensitive to propylene glycol should avoid E430-E436. It has the potential to cause cancer and needs more study. It is banned in some countries. Listed for UK and EU. Not listed for AU, NZ,

Fatty Acid derivatives). Emulsifier(mixing agent), Thickener.	USA and CAN.
E435 **Polysorbate 60** (Emulsifiers and Stabilizers - Fatty Acid derivatives). Emulsifier(mixing agent), Thickener.	$C24H46O6.(C2H4O)n$ It is a synthetic compound that is made from ethylene oxide, sorbitol and stearic acid. Acceptable daily intake is up to 25 mg/kg of body weight.. No noticeable bad effect in concentrations used for most people. People sensitive to propylene glycol should avoid E430-E436. It has the potential to cause cancer and needs more study. Listed for UK, AU, NZ, EU, USA and CAN.
E436 **Polysorbate 65** (Emulsifiers and Stabilizers - Fatty Acid derivatives). Emulsifier(mixing agent), Stabilizer, Anti foaming	It is a synthetic compound that is made from ethylene oxide, sorbitol and stearic acid. Acceptable daily intake is up to 25 mg/kg of body weight. It is used in many products including bakery goods, vegetable oil and in aerosol sprays No noticeable bad effect in concentrations used for most people. People sensitive to propylene glycol should avoid E430-E436. It has the potential to cause cancer and needs more study. Listed for UK, EU, USA and CAN.

agent.	
E440(a) **Pectin.** Thickener, Gelling agent, Stabilizer.	$C_6H_{12}O_6$ It is extracted from citrus fruits, and used in food as a gelling agent particularly in jams and jellies Used in many products including jellies, jams, fillings, sweets, dairy-based desserts, puddings, fruit yogut or flavored yogurt, dairy-based drinks, sauces, condiments, beer, ciders, wines in fruit juices, and a fat substitute in baked goods, many others. Also used as a source of dietary fiber. Typical levels of pectin used as a food additive are between 0.5 – 1.0% - this is about the same amount of pectin as in fresh fruit. Large quantities may cause temporary flatulence or intestinal discomfort. Considered safe in proper usage. Listed for UK, AU, NZ, EU, USA and CAN.
E440(b) **Amidated pectin.** Thickener, Gelling agent, Stabilizer.	Amidated pectin is made by treating pectin with ammonia, see E440(b). No known adverse effects in sources for pectin. Excess However excess ammonia is toxic. Ammonia is a product of protein catabolism and is safely removed by the by the liver. Normal blood ammonia levels range from 10-40 µmol/L. This increases 10% with exposure to 25 ppm, but is not considered harmful. People with

	liver dysfunction may be at increased risk for ammonia toxicity. Listed for UK, USA and EU. Not listed for CAN, AU and NZ.
E441 **Gelatin.** Thickener, Gelling agent, Stabilizer.	$C_6H_{12}O_6$ It is made from the collagen from animal skin and bones. It forms a colorless, nearly tasteless, translucent solid substance that is used as a gelling agent in foods. Gelatin melts when heated, and has a semi-solid form when cooled. It is no longer considered a food additive and is now considered a food. It is commonly used as a gelling agent in foods, such as jellies, jams, yogurt, cream cheese, and margarine, confectionary and for pharmaceuticals (such as "Gel Caps"), and cosmetics. May contain E220 (sulfur dioxide), asthmatics and people allergic to sulfites should be careful. Generally safe, but this is dependent on clean manufacturing processes. You may choose vegetarian gelatin products such as Agar-Agar which is made from seaweed. Often common gelatin is made from pigs. Not listed for UK, EU, AU and NZ. Listed for USA and CAN.
E442	It is a mix of ammonium salts of phosphorylated glycerides and can be

Ammonium phosphatide s. Emulsifier, Stabilizer.	either made synthetically or from mixture of glycerol and partially hardened plant oils. The most often used plant oil in production is Rapeseed oil. But may be made from animal fat including pigs. Used in food industry as an emulsifier, often as an alternative to lecithin. Commonly used in chocolate products and cocoa. No known direct adverse effects. Those with history of heart disease should avoid it in excess as it may clog arteries and heart, like any other altered oil or fat product. This depends on personal genetics. Excess ammonia is toxic, but naturally found in the body as it is a product of protein catabolism and is safely removed by the by the liver. Normal blood ammonia levels range from 10-40 µmol/L. This increases to 10% with exposure to 25 ppm, but is not considered harmful. People with liver dysfunction may be at increased risk for ammonia toxicity. Early symptoms of ammonia toxicity related to decreasing liver function include inability to concentrate, sleepiness and being prone to irritability. Listed for UK, AU, NZ and EU. Not listed for CAN and USA.
E443	It is a vegetable oil that has had

Brominated vegetable oil. (BVO). Emulsifier, Stabilizer.	atoms of the element bromine bonded to it. Brominated vegetable oil is used as an emulsifier in citrus-flavored soft drinks to help natural fat-soluble citrus flavors stay suspended in the drink and to produce a cloudy appearance. BVO has been used by the soft drink industry since 1931. Used in citrus-flavored soft drinks. In the U.S., it has limited use, only in fruit-flavored beverages up to 15 parts per million. Normally safe enough for the vast majority of people. But citrus soft drinks or popular citrus sports drinks or citrus energy drinks taken in excess can cause health problems. "A case reported that a man who consumed two to four liters of a cola containing BVO on a daily basis experienced memory loss, tremors, fatigue, loss of muscle coordination, headache, ptosis of the right eyelid as well as elevated serum chloride. In the two months it took to correctly diagnose the problem, the patient also lost the ability to walk. Eventually bromism was diagnosed and hemodialysis was prescribed which resulted in a reversal of the disorder". Source is Wikipedia. http://en.wikipedia.org/wiki/Brominated_vegetable_oil

	Not listed for UK, AU, NZ and EU. Listed for USA and CAN.
E444 **Sucrose acetate isobutyrate.** Emulsifier, Stabilizer.	$C_{40}H_{62}O_{19}$ Sucrose acetate isobutyrate is a high purity sucrose acetate that is made by the esterification of natural sucrose. It is a tasteless light yellow, highly viscous liquid, used as a stabilizer, and emulsifier in drinks. It can change the density and cloudiness of soft drinks. No bad effects noted in sources. Listed for UK, AU, NZ, EU, USA and CAN.
E445 **Glycerol esters of wood rosins.** Emulsifier, Stabilizer.	Glycerol esters of wood rosin are made by processing wood rosin from the stumps of the longleaf pine. The wood rosin is extracted by solvent extraction, and refined to form an ester gum. It is used as an emulsifier in beverages, to keep oil in suspension. Glycerol ester of wood rosin serves as a natural alternative to brominated vegetable oil in citrus-flavored soft drinks, citrus energy drinks, and citrus sports drinks. High intake over time may upset the calcium/phosphate equilibrium, therefore causing headaches, high blood sugar levels, nausea, vomiting, dehydration, diarrhea, thirst, dizziness, eye, skin irritation and mental confusion. In addition possible adverse reaction for

	sensitive individuals with small amounts. Listed for UK, NZ, AU, EU, USA and CAN.
E446 **Succistearin** . Emulsifier, Stabilizer.	C25 H46 O6 It is produced by the reaction of succinic anhydride, propylene glycol, and hydrogenated vegetable oil. Used as an emulsifier in shortenings and edible oils, to help improve the tenderness in baked goods and bakery items. It is in cakes, cake mixes fillings, icings etc. It breaks down into Propylene glycol-E1520 and fatty acids. Propylene glycol is used to make automobile anti freeze and is a poison. The fatty acids are made up of harmful hydrogenated oil (oil where hydrogen is forced into it at high pressure and heat, which makes so it will not rot or break down easily). Hydrogenated oil is difficult for the body to digest and may cause clogged arteries and other health problems depending on individual genetics. Not listed for UK, EU, AU, NZ and CAN. Listed for USA.
E450 **Sodium and potassium pyrophosph ates.**	Sodium and potassium pyrophosphates are the salts of sodium, calcium and potassium with phosphates. All are produced synthetically and are emulsifying salts. High intakes may upset the

(Diphosphates (two phosphate salt groups put together)). (Mineral salts). **1. Disodium diphosphate** **2.Trisodium diphosphate** **3.Tetrasodium diphosphate** **4. Dipotassium diphosphate** **5.Tetrapotassium diphosphate** **6.Dicalcium diphosphate** **7.Calcium dihydrogen diphosphate** **Emulsifier.** Stabilizer,	digestion and may imbalance the calcium/phosphate equilibrium, IE the body's balance of minerals, or upset the body's digestive enzymes. These mineral salts are used as a buffer and emulsifier, mostly in bread. Linked to kidney stones in sensitive people. Considered safe enough for most people with occasional intake, because proper industrial usage has low concentrations. #6, #7. Mainly used in baked goods, in some calcium supplements etc. Listed for UK, NZ, AU and EU. Not listed for USA and CAN.

Buffer.	
E450(a) **Ammonium phosphate, diabasic and monobasic.** Flour treatment agent, Raising agent, Firming agent, Acidity regulator.	NH4H2PO4 Mineral salt and buffer used with baking powders and salt substitutes. Monobasic Ammonium phosphate is used in baking powder, baked good and bakery products, condiments and desserts. Dibasic Ammonium phosphate is used in baked goods, alcoholic beverages, condiments and desserts. High intakes may upset the digestion, and may imbalance the calcium/phosphate equilibrium, IE the body's balance of minerals, or upset the body's digestive enzymes. Excess ammonia is toxic, but naturally found in the body as it is a product of protein catabolism and is safely removed by the by the liver. Normal blood ammonia levels range from 10-40 µmol/L. This increases to 10% with exposure to 25 ppm, but not considered harmful. People with liver dysfunction may be at increased risk for ammonia toxicity. Early symptoms of ammonia toxicity related to decreasing liver function include inability to concentrate, sleepiness and being prone to irritability. Listed for EU, USA and CAN. Not listed for UK, AU and NZ.
E451	Sodium and potassium salts of phosphoric acid are water-retaining

Sodium and potassium Triphosphate. (Mineral salt). Emulsifier, Stabilizer, Buffer.	agents. Used in bread making to promote the growth of yeast. Considered safe in correct usage, but in large quantities they are known to cause nausea, diarrhea, lowering of blood pressure, cyanosis (blue skin due to lack of oxygen) and muscle spasms. High concentrations of phosphates may disturb several metabolic processes as phosphate plays an important role in general metabolism. Listed for UK, AU, NZ and EU. Not listed for CAN and USA.
E452 **Polyphosphates.** (Mineral salts). **1. Sodium polyphosphate** **2. Potassium polyphosphate** **3. Sodium calcium** **polyphosphate** **4. Calcium**	Salts of sodium, potassium, calcium, and ammonium with phosphate, are produced synthetically with carbonates and phosphoric acid. Used as sequestrants (metal binders), stabilizers and emulsifiers. Used in cupcake mixes, instant pasta and sauces and ice-cream. Phosphates are involved in many body processes and higher than normal concentrations can cause health problems. Linked to kidney stones in susceptible people, otherwise regarded as safe. Caution See 338 Excess ammonia is toxic, however it is naturally found in the body as it is a product of protein catabolism and is safely removed by the by the liver. Normal blood

polyphosph ate **5.** **Ammonium polyphosph ate.** Emulsifier, Stabilizer, Sequestrant(b inding agent).	ammonia levels range from 10-40 μmol/L. This increases 10% with exposure to 25 ppm, but is not considered harmful. People with liver dysfunction may be at increased risk for ammonia toxicity. Some early symptoms of ammonia toxicity related to decreasing liver function include inability to concentrate, sleepiness and being prone to irritability. Listed for UK, AU, NZ and EU. Not listed for CAN and USA.
E459 **Beta-cyclodextrin e.** Anti Oxidant, Emulsifier (mixing agent), Stabilizer.	Made from starch by the use of enzymatic conversion. Can turn liquid food into solid food. It has a ring (donut) structure, so it can bind other molecules into the center of it, giving it special useful properties. For instance, it can remove the bitter taste or bad smell from a tainted food. Used in spices, cereal, chewing gum, and in canned fruit drinks. No known bad effects listed in sources. Listed for EU and UK. Not listed for AU, NZ, CAN and USA.
E460 **Cellulose.** (Cellulose and derivatives). Anti-caking agent,	$(C_6H_{10}O_5)_n$ Cellulose is mostly the cell walls of green plants and algae; it can be made from cotton (source cotton may be genetically modified) and wood. Can be in soup, breads, biscuits and cakes, frozen desserts, sauces, cream, crisps, spreads, jams, chocolate,

Emulsifier(mixing agent), Thickener, Dietary fiber.	margarine, deserts, and milk shakes. An anti-caking agent and base for solid tablets, no adverse effects known in proper usage, but provides no nutrition. Cellulose is non soluble, so won't dissolve in water, but can be fermented in the large intestine. Large concentrations can cause intestinal problems, such as bloating and constipation, caution for those with digestion problems. Caution with small children and babies because it is difficult to digest, especially in concentration. Banned in UK for baby food. Listed for UK, AU, NZ, EU, USA and CAN.
E461 **Methylcellulose.** (Cellulose and derivatives). Emulsifier(mixing agent), Thickener.	It is mainly made up of the cell walls of green plants and algae. Commercially it is usually made from wood and cotton (source cotton may be genetically modified) by heating the cellulose with a caustic solution and treating it with methyl chloride. It produces a hydrophilic (water loving) powder that when dissolved forms a clear viscous gel. Used in low-calorie cream, ice cream, toothpaste and laxatives. Caution, can cause flatulence, distension, and intestinal obstruction especially in excess. Listed for UK, AU, NZ, EU, USA and CAN.
E462	Emulsifier (mixing agent), thickener

Ethyl cellulose Cellulose and derivatives	is similar to E461, see above, but rarely used. Can be used as a thin-film coating material on foods. Listed for EU, UK and USA. Not listed for AU, NZ and CAN.
E463 **Hydroxypro pyl cellulose.** (Cellulose and derivatives). Emulsifier(mixing agent), Thickener, Dietary fiber.	C_3H_7O It can be made from cotton (source cotton may be genetically modified) and wood. Similar to cellulose, but more soluble in water. Used in pasteurized products, ice-creams, cheeses, dairy products, batters, spreads, breakfast cereals, and baked goods etc. It is fairly soluble, and can be fermented in the large intestine. Large concentrations can cause bloating, constipation and diarrhea. May be used in eye medications, be careful of adverse reactions, consult your doctor. In concentration can be toxic to lungs, eyes and skin. Not listed for AU. Listed for UK, NZ, AU, USA, EU and CAN.
E464 **Hydroxypro pyl-Methylcellul ose.** (Cellulose and derivatives). Emulsifier(mi	Similar as E463, but more soluble in water, it is under study to use as a replacement for gluten in bread. A vegetarian substitute for gelatin, it is slightly more expensive to produce due to a semi synthetic manufacturing processes. Listed for UK, NZ, AU, EU and CAN. Not listed for USA.

xing agent), Thickener, Dietary fiber.	
E465 **Methyl ethyl cellulose or Ethylmethyl cellulose.** (Cellulose and derivatives). Emulsifier(mixing agent), Stabilizer, Foaming agent.	It is made from cellulose (source cotton may be genetically modified) then chemically modified. Mainly a thickening agent, but also used as a filler, dietary fiber, anti clumping, and emulsifying agent Similar to cellulose E460, common uses include ice-creams, cheeses, dairy products, batters, baked emulsions, spreads, breakfast cereals, and baked goods. Methyl ethyl cellulose is not very water soluble, and can be fermented in the large intestine. Large concentrations can cause intestinal problems, such as bloating, constipation and diarrhea. Listed for UK, NZ, AU, EU, USA and CAN.
E466 **Carboxymethyl cellulose or Sodium carboxymethyl cellulose or Carboxymethylcellulose.** (Cellulose and derivatives).	It is made from cellulose (source cotton may be genetically modified) then chemically modified with chloroacetic acid. Mainly a thickening agent, but also used as a filler, dietary fiber, anti clumping and emulsifying agent. Similar to cellulose-E460, common uses include pasteurized products, ice-creams, cheeses, dairy products, batters, baked emulsions, spreads, breakfast cereals, and baked goods. It is very water soluble. Known to cause

Emulsifier(mixing agent), Thickener.	cancer in test animals, caution. Large amounts can be fermented in the large intestine. Large concentrations can cause intestinal problems, such as gas, bloating, constipation and diarrhea Listed for UK, NZ, AU, USA, EU and CAN.
E467 **Ethyl hydroxyethyl cellulose.** (Cellulose and derivatives). Emulsifier(mixing agent), Thickener, Stabilizer.	It is a semi-synthetic polysaccharide with its primary component being the cell walls of green plants and algae. Industrially it can be made from wood and chemically modified by treatment with alkali, ethylene oxide, and ethyl chloride. It is used in dairy-based drinks, processed cheese, fat spreads, processed fruits, confectionary, baked goods, batters, condiments, processed meats, beer and wine. Also used in soaps and cleaning products, can be used as a laxative. Not much information on safety. What little information shows it is not very toxic in small amounts with test animals, but adverse effects found with a higher amounts. Not listed for UK, CAN, NZ, AU, USA and EU. http://www.inchem.org/documents/jecfa/jecmono/v26je08.htm
E468 **Crosslinked**	Produced by acidifying sodium carboxymethyl cellulose E466 (source cotton may be genetically

sodium carboxymet hyl cellulose or Croscarmell ose sodium. Emulsifier (mixing agent), Stabilizers.	modified) and heating it until the suspension is able to achieve cross-linking. The cross-linking reduces water solubility while still allowing the material to swell (like a sponge) and absorb many times its weight in water. As a result, it provides superior drug dissolution (ability to go into solution) and disintegration characteristics for medicines. Used in pasteurized products, ice-creams, cheeses, dairy products, batters, baked emulsions and spreads, breakfast cereals, and baked goods etc. Not much information on safety either way. See E466. Listed for UK, EU. Not listed for NZ, AU, CAN and USA. http://ec.europa.eu/food/fs/sc/scf/o ut02_en.html
E469 **Sodium caseinate or Casein.** Emulsifiers (mixing agent), Stabilizers.	It is a emulsifier and mineral salt made from casein in cow's milk. Used for thickener, beverage whitener in dessert mixes and reduced cream whip. People with milk allergy should avoid. It may improve some people's mental ability and health when avoided, some studies indicate that avoiding casein products helps with autistic and learning impaired children. Similar consideration with products with gluten in them. If allergic to any one

	of these-milk products, casein or gluten, may be allergic to all, also consider lectin allergy. Casein may impair mental and or physical function and health, it may increase cancer growth, may cause cancer. Sometimes negative effects may be slight with little acute noticeable allergies or adverse reactions, and if so it is difficult to determine cause and effect, the effect often increases with age and becomes noticeable. Not listed for AU, NZ and CAN. Listed for USA. (Note, it appears that there are two additives with E number E469 in common usage, depending on the country)
E469 **Enzymatical ly hydrolyzed carboxymet hyl cellulose.** Emulsifier(mi xing agent), Stabilizers.	It is the sodium salt of carboxymethyl ether of cellulose, hydrolyzed enzymatically with Trichoderma Longibrachiatum. Primarily it is used as a stabilizer with fat-extending properties. Used in soft drinks, as a whitener, and in low-fat and reduced fat foods, cream, cheeses, spreads, and dairy based desserts. No adverse effects noted in sources. Listed for UK and EU. Not listed for CAN and USA.
E470(a) **Sodium, Potassium**	Sodium, potassium and calcium salts of fatty acids, mainly from plant origin, but also fats of animal origin may be used, including pork. The

and Calcium Salts of Fatty Acids. (Salt or Ester of Fatty Acid). Emulsifier (mixing agent), Stabilizer.	body metabolizes the products as any other fat, it can cause gastric upset. These are unnatural fats, caution, may be toxic, especially if eaten in excess over time. Banned in some countries. Listed for UK, NZ, AU, EU and USA. Not listed for CAN.
E470(b) **Magnesium salts of fatty acids, also Al, Ca, Na, K and NH4.** (Salt or Ester of Fatty Acid). Emulsifier (mixing agent), Stabilizer.	Similar as E470(a). Particular caution with fatty salts with ammonia and aluminum, both in excess may cause health problems, but generally not harmful for most people in slight trace amounts. Listed for UK, NZ, AU, EU, USA and CAN.
E471 **Mono-and Diglycerides of Fatty Acids.** (Salt or Ester of Fatty Acid).	Made from glycerol and natural fatty acids, primarily from hydrogenated soya bean oil but may be animal based, possibly pig fat. Can be used in whipped cream, ice-cream, cakes, baked goods, dairy foods, dehydrated potatoes, hot-chocolate mix, etc. May contain trans fats, no known direct adverse effects, but

Emulsifier (mixing agent), Stabilizer.	may be harmful to arteries and heart if trans fats are eaten in excess over many months to years. Caution, especially if you have a family history of heart disease. Listed for UK, NZ, AU, EU, USA and CAN.
E472a **Acetic and fatty acid esters of glycerol.** (Salt or Ester of Fatty Acid). Emulsifier (mixing agent), Stabilizer.	Esters of mono- and diglycerides of fatty acids are produced from glycerol, natural fatty acids, and acetic acid. The origin of the fatty acids is mainly from plants, but may also come from animals-pigs. Caution, in rare cases may cause diarrhea, thirst, dizziness and mental confusion for sensitive people. Used as a coating on meats, nuts and fruits to extend shelf life. Also used in whipped products and fats, dairy-based drinks, batters, yogurts, edible ices, breakfast cereals etc. Not more than 2mg/Kg. Caution with excessive usage of any kind of unnatural fat. Listed for UK, AU, NZ and EU. Not listed for USA and CAN.
E472b **Lactic and fatty acid esters of glycerol.** (Salt or Ester of Fatty Acid).	It is made from glycerol, natural fatty acids, and lactic acid. Usually plant based, but may be made from animal fat-pig fat. Also used as a coating agent, texture modifier, solvent and lubricant. May cause some people to have diarrhea, thirst, dizziness and mental confusion. Can be in bakery products, breakfast cereals, whipped

Emulsifier (mixing agent), Stabilizer.	products and fats, dairy-based drinks, yogurts, batters, etc. Caution with excessive usage of any kind of unnatural fat. Listed for UK, AU, NZ, EU, USA and CAN.
E472 c **Citric and fatty acid esters of glycerol.** (Salt or Ester of Fatty Acid). Emulsifier (mixing agent), Stabilizer.	It is made from glycerol, natural fatty acids, and citric acid. Usually plant based, but may be made from animal fat-pig fat. May cause some people to have diarrhea, thirst, dizziness and mental confusion. Used in baked products, whipped products and in fats. Caution with excessive usage of any kind of unnatural fat. Listed for UK, AU, NZ, USA and EU. Not listed for CAN. http://www.accessdata.fda.gov/scripts/fcn/gras_notices/grn000222.pdf
E472d **Tartaric acid esters of monoglyceri des and diglycerides of fatty acids.** (Salt or Ester of Fatty Acid). Emulsifier	It is made from glycerol, natural fatty acids, and tartaric acid. Usually plant based, but may be made from animal fat-pig fat. May cause some people to have diarrhea, thirst, dizziness and mental confusion Used in baked products, whipped products and in fats. Caution with excessive usage of any kind of unnatural fat. Listed for UK and EU. Not listed for USA, AU, NZ and CAN.

(mixing agent), Stabilizer.	
E472e **Mono and diacetyl tartaric acid esters of mono and diglycerides of fatty acids.** (Salt or Ester of Fatty Acid). Emulsifier (mixing agent), Stabilizer.	Made from glycerol, natural fatty acids, and diacetyl tartaric acid. Usually plant based, but may be made from animal fat-pig fat. Used in baked products, whipped products and in fats. In sensitive people may cause headaches, high blood sugar levels, and eye/skin irritation. Caution with excessive usage of any kind of unnatural fat. Listed for UK, AU, NZ and EU. Not listed for CAN and USA.
E472f **Mixed acetic and tartaric acid esters of mono- and diglycerides of fatty acids.** (Salt or Ester of Fatty Acid).	Made from glycerol, natural fatty acids, acetic, and tartaric acids. Usually plant based, but may be made from animal fat-pig fat. May cause some people to have diarrhea, thirst, dizziness and mental confusion. Can be in baked products, whipped products and fats, dairy-based drinks, yoghurts, , batters, breakfast cereals, edible ices, etc. Caution with excessive usage of any kind of unnatural fat. Listed for UK, NZ, AU and EU. Not listed for CAN

Emulsifier (mixing agent), Stabilizer.	and USA.
E473 **Sucrose Esters of Fatty Acids.** (Salt or Ester of Fatty Acid). Emulsifier (mixing agent), Stabilizer.	The mono, di and triesters of sucrose with edible fatty acids, and are made by use of solvents. Usually plant based, but may be made from animal fat-pig fat. It may have traces of solvents. The body metabolizes all components identical to sugar and natural fat. May cause stomach pain, nausea, bloating, diarrhea in sensitive people. Used to stabilize soups, dairy desserts, mayonnaise and margarine. May be in chewing gum, coffee and tea beverages with added dairy ingredients, may be used as a protective coating on fresh fruit. Listed for UK, NZ, AU and EU. Not listed for CAN and USA.
E474 **Sucroglycer ides.** (Salt or Ester of Fatty Acid). Emulsifier (mixing agent), Stabilizer.	It is made by reacting sucrose and fat/oil together with or without the presence of a solvent. Usually fat is plant based (can be from genetically modified plants), but may be made from animal fat-pig fat. Usually the solvent is either dimethyl formamide, cyclohexane, isobutanol, isopropanol, or ethyl acetate. Used in chewing gum, cereals, heat treated meat, fruit based desserts, cocoa mixes, dairy based drinks, dairy

	based desserts weight reduction formulae, and electrolyte drinks. Not used in Australia, caution, best to avoid. Listed for UK, EU. Not listed for AU, NZ, CAN and USA.
E475 **Polyglycerol Esters of Fatty Acids.** (Salt or Ester of Fatty Acid). Emulsifier (mixing agent), Stabilizer.	It is made by the combination of polyglycerol, and natural fats derived from soybean, rapeseed and maize (any of these can be genetically modified). Usually source fat is plant based, but may be made from animal fat-pig fat. May be in milk powder for baby formula, imitation milk powders, icings, coffee whitener, bakery and pastry products, chewing gum, butter, and cake mixes. No known direct adverse effects. Caution with excessive usage of any kind of unnatural fat. Listed for UK, NZ, AU, EU, USA and CAN.
E476 **Polyglycerol esters of interesterifi ed ricinoliec acid,** **or** **Polyglycerol polyricinole ate.** (Salt or Ester of Fatty Acid).	It is made from the combination of polyglycerol, and castor oil. It improves fluidity of some liquids especially chocolate, and also enables coatings to be thinly spread, like spreads and salad dressings. Acceptable Daily Intake: Up to 7.5 mg/kg bodyweight. No known direct adverse effects. Caution with excessive usage of any kind of unnatural fat. Listed for UK, NZ, AU, EU and CAN. Not listed for USA.

Emulsifier (mixing agent), Stabilizer.	
E477 **Propylene glycol mono-esters and di-esters of fatty acids.** (Salt or Ester of Fatty Acid). Emulsifier (mixing agent), Stabilizer.	It is made by the esterification or transesterification of propylene glycol and fatty acids. Usually source fat is plant based (can be from genetically modified plants), but may be made from animal fat-pig fat. In baked products, soft drinks, ice-cream, and processed meats, etc. Caution, propylene glycol is the principle ingredient of auto antifreeze and is toxic. Propylene glycol is poison, can cause nervous system damage, kidney damage, harm vision and eyes etc. Some people more sensitive than others, avoid it. Especially avoid if have kidney or liver impairment. Listed for UK, NZ, AU, EU, USA and CAN.
E478 **Lactylated fatty acid esters of glycerol and propane-1, 2-diol.** (Salt or Ester of Fatty Acid).	It is made from the reaction of propylene glucol ester with lactic acid, propanediol, and natural fats. Usually source fat is plant based (can be from genetically modified plants), but may be made from animal fat-pig fat. Used in products that need aeration such as toppings, cake mixes, and coffee whitener. May cause headaches, nausea, vomiting,

Emulsifier (mixing agent), Stabilizer.	dehydration, diarrhea, thirst, dizziness and mental confusion. Best to avoid. Not listed for EU, UK, NZ, AU and CAN. Listed for USA.
E479b **Esterified soy oil.** (Salt or Ester of Fatty Acid). Emulsifier (mixing agent), Stabilizer.	It is thermally oxidized soy bean oil that is mixed with mono- and diglycerides of fatty acids. Usually source fat is plant based (may be genetically modified), but may be made from animal fat-pig fat. Used in baked products. Caution with excessive usage of any kind of unnatural fats. Listed for UK and EU. Not listed for AU, NZ, CAN and USA.
E480 **Dioctyl sodium sulphosuccinate.** Emulsifier (mixing agent), Stabilizer.	$C24H38O4$ It is made by the reaction of octane with maleic acid anhydride, followed by the reaction with sodium ⬜ sulfate. Used in bakery goods, dairy products, chewing gum, and soft drinks. Waiting for study results especially in regards with small children. Caution. Not listed for UK and EU. Listed for AU, NZ, CAN and USA.
E481 **Sodium Stearoyl-2-Lactylate.**	$C21H39NaO4$ It is made by combining stearic acid and lactic acid, with sodium hydroxide. Flour treatment stabilizer, emulsifier to make it able to retain

Emulsifier (mixing agent), Stabilizer.	shape after going through machinery. Used in baked goods, whipping agents, salad dressings, soups, and non dairy creamers. No known bad effects listed in sources. Listed for UK, NZ, AU, EU, USA and CAN.
E482 **Calcium Stearoyl Lactylate.** Emulsifier (mixing agent), Stabilizer.	C42H78CaO8 It is made by combining stearic acid and lactic acid with calcium hydroxide, ending up with a calcium salt. Used in baked goods, whipping agents, salad dressings, soups, and non dairy creamers. No known bad effects listed in sources for people. But some animal tests have shown adverse reactions, caution. Listed for UK, NZ, AU, EU and USA. Not listed for CAN.
E483 **Stearyl Tartrate.** Emulsifier (mixing agent), Stabilizer.	C40H78O6 It is made by the esterification of tartaric acid with stearyl alcohol. Used in baked products. May cause cancer? Banned in Australia, and other countries, extreme caution. Listed for UK and EU. Not listed for AU, NZ, CAN and USA.
E484 **Stearyl citrate.**	It is made by the esterification of citric acid with stearyl alcohol. The stearyl acid can be made from either plant or animal fat, more often plant based and source plants may be

Emulsifier (mixing agent), Sequestrant (binding agent).	genetically modified and the source fat may be made from hydrogenated oil. Used in baked goods. No information on safety either way in sources. Not listed for UK, NZ, AU, EU and CAN. Listed for USA.
E485 **Sodium stearyl fumarate.** Emulsifier (mixing agent), Flour treatment agent.	$C22H39NaO4$ Sodium stearoyl fumarate is an organic compound made by combining stearic acid and fumaric acid with sodium hydroxide. The stearyl acid can be made from either plant or animal fat, more often plant based and source plants may be genetically modified and may be made from hydrogenated oil. Used in baked goods. No information on safety either way in sources. Not listed for UK, AU, NZ, EU. Listed for CAN and USA.
E486 **Calcium stearyl fumarate.** Emulsifier (mixing agent), Flour treatment agent.	It is made by combining stearic acid and fumaric acid, with calcium hydroxide. The stearyl acid can be made from either plant or animal fat, more often plant based and source plants may be genetically modified and may be made from hydrogenated oil. Used in baked goods and dehydrated potatoes. No information on safety either way in sources. Not listed for UK, AU, NZ, EU, USA and CAN.
E487	$C12H25NaO4S$

Sodium lauryl sulfate Emulsifier (mixing agent), Thickener.	It is industrially synthesized from sulfuric acid as sulfuric acid monododecyl ester sodium salt, or naturally from coconut and/or palm oil kernels. Used in egg whites, marshmallows, fruit juices, fats and oils. Skin contact may have adverse reactions, moderately toxic when ingested, may be mutagenic, caution. Not listed for UK, NZ, AU and EU. Listed for CAN and USA.
E488 **Ethoxylated Mono- and Di-Glycerides.** Emulsifier(mixing agent), Raising agent, Flour treatment agent.	They are made by glycerolysis of edible fats, primarily composed of stearic, palmitic, and myristic acids, or direct esterification of glycerol with a mixture of primarily stearic, palmitic and myristic acids. Used as an emulsifier in pan-release agents, cakes and cake mixes, whipped vegetable oil toppings and topping mixes, icings and icing mixes, frozen desserts, edible vegetable fat emulsions, intended for use as substitutes for milk or cream in coffee. Excess ingestion may result in gastric disturbances. No information in sources about safety. Not listed for UK, EU, NZ, AU and CAN. Listed for USA. http://blog.caloricious.com/2011/06/03/ethoxylated-mono-and-diglycerides-e488-emulsifier-and-dough-conditioner/

E489 **Methyl glucoside - Coconut oil ester.** Emulsifier(mixing agent), Humectant (water retaining agent), Surfactant (lowers liquid surface tension to aid mixing), Flavoring agent.	It is an organic compound made from coconut oil. Used for the dehydration of grapes to produce raisins, crystallization of sucrose, and as a synthetic flavoring agent. As a surfactant in molasses at a level not to exceed 320 parts per million (USA). No information in sources about safety. Caution with excessive usage of any kind of unnatural fats. Not listed for NZ, UK, AU, EU and CAN. Listed for USA.
E490 **Propane-1,2-diol or Propylene glycol.** Emulsifier, (mixing agent), Stabilizer, Humectant	$C_3H_8O_2$ It is also known as propylene glycol, is an organic compound that is commercially produced by the hydration of propylene oxide, but can also be derived from glycerol. Used in margarine, baked goods, seasonings, alcoholic beverages, flavorings, frostings, cold dairy products, confectionary, chocolates, sweetened coconut, chewing gum, pre prepared food and nut products and it is a carrier liquid for food colors and

(water retaining agent), Anti-microbial.	flavorings. It can cause nervous system damage and kidney damage. It is a primary ingredient in automobile anti-freeze, a serious poison that should be kept away from children and pets (they may drink because it can be slightly sweet in taste). Those who are sensitive or with impaired kidney/liver function should have extra caution. I personally had a kidney pain attack from toothpaste, with propylene glycol as an ingredient. Not listed for UK, AU, NZ and EU. Listed for CAN and USA.
E491 **Sorbitan monosteara te.** Emulsifier (mixing agent) Stabilizer, Defoaming agent, Flavor dispersing agent.	$C_{24}H_{46}O_6$ It is made from an ester of sorbitan and stearic acid. It produces a waxy-like cream powder that is very soluble in water. Used primarily as an emulsifier in cake mixes, imitation whipped cream, baked goods, and puddings. No known quick bad effects for humans but in some animal studies shown to cause growth retardation and may cause bile duct changes in the liver. May be made from soy or peanuts and from genetically modified plants, may contain trace amounts of 1, 4-dioxane, which is a cancer causing agent. Listed for UK, AU, NZ, EU, USA and CAN.

E492 **Sorbitan tristearate.** Emulsifier (mixing agent), Stabilizer, Surfactant (lowers liquid surface tension).	$C_{60}H_{114}O_8$ It is made from an ester of sorbitan and stearic acid. It produces a waxy-like cream powder that is soluble in hot water. Only allowed in "compounded chocolate" (a cheaper chocolate product made from a combination of cocoa, vegetable fat, and sweeteners) that is used in chocolate and cake mixes.. May increase the absorption of liquid paraffin and fat-soluble substances. May be made from soy or peanuts, may be made from genetically modified plants, may contain trace amounts of 1, 4- dioxane, which is a cancer causing agent, caution. Listed for UK, AU, NZ, EU and CAN. Not listed for USA.
E493 **Sorbitan monolaurate.** (Salts or Esters of Fatty Acids). Emulsifier (mixing agent), Stabilizer.	C18H34O6 It is made from the mixture of partial esters of sorbitol, and mono- and dianhydrides with lauric acid, a natural fatty acid derived from plant or animal origin. Emulsifier and stabilizer, it stops sugar mixes from foaming. May be made from soy or peanuts, may be made from genetically modified plants, it may contain trace amounts of 1, 4- dioxane, which is a cancer causing agent. Not listed for USA, AU, NZ and others. Listed for UK and EU.

E494	C24H44O6
Sorbitan mono-oleate. (Salts or Esters of Fatty Acids). Emulsifier (mixing agent), Stabilizer.	It is made from the mixture of partial esters of sorbitol, and its mono- and dianhydrides with oleic acid a natural fatty acid derived from plant or animal origin. Used in ice cream, yeast products and pharmaceuticals. May be made from soy or peanuts, may be made from genetically modified plants, it may contain trace amounts of 1, 4- dioxane, which is a cancer causing agent. Listed for UK, EU and USA. Not listed for CAN, NZ and AU.
E495 **Sorbitan monopalmitate.** (Salts or Esters of Fatty Acids). Emulsifier (mixing agent), Stabilizer.	C22H42O6 It is made from the mixture of partial esters of sorbitol and its mono- and dianhydrides with palmitic acid a natural fatty acid. Used in many kinds of products. It may be made from soy or peanuts, may be made from genetically modified plants, may contain trace amounts of 1, 4- dioxane, which is a cancer causing agent. Banned in Australia and others, avoid it. Listed for UK and EU. Not listed for NZ, AU, CAN and USA.
E496 **Sorbitan trioleat.** (Salts or	It is a polysorbate that is derived from the mixture of partial tri-esters of sorbitol, no known common uses. May be made from soy or peanuts, may be made from genetically

Esters of Fatty Acids). Emulsifier (mixing agent), Stabilizer.	modified plants, may contain trace amounts of 1, 4- dioxane, which is a cancer causing agent. Not listed for UK, NZ, AU, EU and USA. Listed for CAN.
E497 **Polyoxypro pylene-polyoxyethy lene polymers.** Surfactant (lowers liquid surface tension), Emulsifier (mixing agent), Stabilizer.	It is salts or esters of fatty acids. Used in milk powders, milk replacements and in feed for animals, which may be eaten by humans. Studied for many medical uses, such as carrying various medicines such as carrying medicines in cancer treatment, but is not inert for body and cellular processes. The study noted below indicates it is safe, but more study is needed. Not listed for UK, AU, NZ, EU and CAN. Listed for USA. http://ec.europa.eu/food/fs/sc/oldc omm6/other/21_en.pdf
E498 **Partial polyglycerol esters of polyconden sed fatty acids of castor oil.** (Salts or Esters of Fatty	It is made by the combination of polyglycerol, and castor oil (the oil from the Ricinus sp tree). Used in cake mixes, chocolate, icings, low-fat spreads, salad dressings, and chocolate. No information about safety found in sources. Not listed for UK, NZ, AU, EU and CAN. Listed for USA.

Acids). Emulsifier (mixing agent), Stabilizer, Surfactant (lowers liquid surface tension).	

Vegetable gums & stabilizers E499-E585:

Vegetable gums may be used as thickening agents. When added into a food mixture they increase viscosity without greatly modifying other properties, such as taste. They provide body, increase stability, and improve suspending properties.

Common examples of gums are agar, alginin, arrowroot, collagen, cornstarch, fecula, gelatin, guar gum, katakuri, locust bean gum, pectin, rehan, roux, tapioca, and xanthan gum.

E499	$(C_6H_{10}O_5)n$
Cassia gum. (Vegetable gums & stabilizers). Emulsifier (mixing agent), Gelling agent.	Made from the endosperm of *Senna obtusifolia* (also called *Cassia obtusifolia* or *Cassia tora*). It is used in pet food, but manufacturers are wanting to expand it into human foods in recent years-2009 onward. It is beneficial for lowering cholesterol, blood pressure and blood sugar. Pregnant women should avoid. Contains coumarin, best to

	avoid large amounts of Cassia gum and potential for adverse reactions for some sensitive people. Listed for UK and EU. Not listed for UK, NZ, AU, USA and CAN.
E500 (Sodium carbonates). **1. Sodium carbonate. (washing soda or soda ash)** **2. Sodium hydrogen carbonate. (Bicarbonat e of soda).** **3. Sodium sesquicarbo nate.** (Vegetable gums & stabilizers). Acidity regulator, Anti-caking agent, Raising agent,	Na_2CO_3 It is the sodium salt of carbonic acid, which is carbon dioxide dissolved in water. It is more commonly known as washing soda or soda ash. It is synthetically produced in large quantities from table salt. Made by the reaction of calcium carbonate, sodium chloride and carbon dioxide in water and ammonia. It is an acidity regulator, particularly important in making beer. Used while making beer, soft drinks, carbonated beverages, noodles, and baked goods, etc. At high amounts may irritate stomach and the fizz can irritate eyes and respiratory track. Some sources indicate that at high amounts it may be a Teratogen: (A agent that can disturb the development of an embryo or fetus). Those with heart problems may consider avoiding, it may cause gastrointestinal problems for some people. No direct adverse effects for most people in proper usage. Listed for UK, AU, NZ EU, USA and CAN.
E501	K_2CO_3

Potassium carbonate. (Vegetable gums & stabilizers). Acidity regulator, Buffering agent.	It is made synthetically for commercial use by the electrolysis of potassium chloride. The resulted potassium hydroxide is then carbonated using carbon dioxide to form potassium carbonate. It is a mineral salt, an adjusting and modifying agent Used as gastric antacid and to replenish electrolytes in the body Used in baked goods, soft drinks cocoa, confectionary, custard powder, cocoa and wine. Similar to E500. Consider avoiding if have kidney or heart problems. No known direct adverse effects for most people in proper usage. Listed for UK, AU, NZ, EU, USA and CAN.
E503 (Ammonium carbonates). **1. Ammoum carbonate.** **2. Ammoni um hydrogen carbonate**. (Vegetable gums & stabilizers).	$(NH_4)_2CO_3$ It is made by heating a mixture of ammonium chloride and chalk. Used in medications, baked goods, baking powder, cocoa, confectionary and ice cream, can be used as smelling salts to revive people. As a leavening agent it makes breads lighter with air pockets inside. A mineral salt, adjusting and modifying agent, it alters the pH of urine and may cause loss of calcium and magnesium. May irritate mucous membranes and lead to skin and scalp irritations in some people. Excess ammonia is toxic, but is naturally inside the body as it

Raising agent for baked goods, Acidy regulator.	is a product of protein catabolism and is safely removed by the by the liver. Normal blood ammonia levels range from 10-40 µmol/L. This increases 10% with exposure to 25 ppm, but is not considered harmful. People with liver dysfunction may be at increased risk for ammonia toxicity. Early symptoms of ammonia toxicity related to decreasing liver function include inability to concentrate, sleepiness and being prone to irritability. Listed for UK, EU, NZ, AU, USA and CAN.
E504 **Magnesium carbonate or Magnesium hydroxide carbonate.** (Vegetable gums & stabilizers). Acidy regulator, Anti-caking agent.	$MgCO_3$ It is made by exposing magnesium hydroxide to carbon dioxide under pressure. Used in sugar, salt and other granular foods, also in whey products, powdered sugar, toothpaste and salt. Used as antiacid, supplement and laxative. Magnesium carbonate, most often referred to as 'chalk', is used as a drying agent, for instance as a white powder for hands in rock climbing, gymnastics, and weight lifting (may be harmful to lungs if breathed in to excess). No known bad effects in normal usage for most people. Ingesting high amounts may have a laxative effect. Those with kidney problems may need to avoid. In general, caution

	with excessive long term usage, months-years-decades of any kind of non food based supplements as it may be hard on organs (kidneys, liver etc). Also be cautious of using any single mineral or vitamin at high dosage for a long time (months-years or longer) as it may throw the body out of balance. Listed for UK, NZ, AU, EU, USA and CAN.
E505 **Ferrous carbonate.** (Fortify foods and Supplement). Acidy regulator.	$FeCO_3$ Precipitated by the result of the reaction of ferrous sulfate and sodium carbonate in an aqueous medium. Used in iron-fortified foods, and iron supplements. Caution with excessive long term usage, months-years-decades of any kind of non food based supplements as it may be hard on organs (kidneys, liver etc). Also be cautious of using any single mineral or vitamin at high dosage for a long time (months-years or longer) as it may throw the body out of balance. Not listed for UK, EU, NZ, AU and CAN. Listed for USA.
E507 **Hydrochloric acid,** **or** **Muriatic acid,**	$HCl+H2O$ It is made by adding gaseous hydrogen chloride to water. The resulting acid is highly corrosive and a strong mineral acid. Hydrochloric acid is found naturally in the stomach. It is used as an acidity

or Chlorohydric acid. Acidy regulator, Acidic in Ph.	regulator in food. May have teratogenic (birth defect) properties and may be carcinogenic when mixed with formaldehyde. Considered safe enough in very small amounts, in proper usage. Concentrated hydrochloric acid is very toxic and corrosive. Listed for UK, AU, NZ, EU, USA and CAN.
E508 **Potassium chloride or** Muriate **of potash.** (Vegetable gums & stabilizers). Gelling agent, Acidity regulator, Thickener. Stabilizer, Supplement.	KCl It is a mineral salt composed of chlorine and potassium, usually extracted from salt water, and can be used in place of salt. May be used as an electrolyte to replace lost potassium. Used in brewing, as a salt substitute for low to zero salt products and as a gelling agent. Can be associated with gastric ulcers, circulatory collapse, nausea, liver toxicity and kidney problems. Extra caution with small children, they may be unable to effectively digest it. Avoid if have heart, kidney or liver problems. It is a non plant based source of potassium, be cautious of excessively using any non plant based supplements long term, months to years as it may be harmful to organs over time. Also long term (months to years to decades) usage of any single mineral supplement in excessive amounts may throw the

	internal body minerals out of balance. Listed for UK, NZ, AU, EU, USA and CAN.
E509 **Calcium chloride.** Sequestrant (binding agent), Firming agent, Preservative.	$CaCl_2$ It is made from limestone, although commercially it can be exacted from sea salt and rock salt (from brine which is salt water). It is a salt, commonly used for road de-icing, it looks like small round balls called prills. Used in jelly, cheese, and to keep canned fruit/vegetable firm. Electrolyte for some sports drinks, pickles and sometimes used in beer making, possible stomach irritant for sensitive people. Considered safe in listed sources. It is the active ingredient in some home use dampness removal products-calcium chloride dust may cause an allergic reaction when breathed. Listed for UK, AU, NZ, EU, USA and CAN.
E510 **Ammonium chloride or Sal ammoniac.** Acidity regulator,	NH_4Cl It is made by reacting ammonia with hydrogen chloride. Used in baked goods, flour products, bread mixes, fermented drinks, and low-sodium salt substitutes. A 5% by weight solution of ammonium chloride in water has a pH in the range 4.6 to 6.0. Sal ammoniac is a name of the natural, mineralogical form of ammonium chloride. People with

Flavor enhancer.	kidney and liver problems should avoid, also children. Large amounts can cause nausea, headaches and insomnia. Excess ammonia is toxic, but found naturally in the body as it is a product of protein catabolism and is safely removed by the by the liver. Normal blood ammonia levels range from 10-40 µmol/L. This increases to 10% with exposure to 25 ppm, but is not considered harmful. People with liver dysfunction may be at increased risk for ammonia toxicity. Early symptoms of ammonia toxicity related to decreasing liver function include inability to concentrate, sleepiness and being prone to irritability. Not listed for UK and EU. Listed for NZ, AU, CAN and USA.
E511 **Magnesium chloride.** Firming agent, Stabilizer, Color retention agent.	$MgCl_2$ It is part of natural salts in sea water. Can be mined out of ancient sea beds or produced from sea water after the sodium chloride is removed. Used in jelly, raw meat cuts, poultry, and artificially sweetened preserves, soy milk and tofu. A good source of magnesium which is an essential mineral, a lack of magnesium is a very common deficiency, but must be in balance with other minerals, too little or too much in relation to other

	minerals can cause health problems. Caution with usage of magnesium chloride if have kidney problems, because excess is excreted in the urine by the kidneys. Best to have any long term (months to years to decades) supplementation to be in balance with all other minerals and to be plant based (to be easier on organs). Generally considered safe in normal usage as an additive. Listed for UK, AU, NZ, EU, USA and CAN.
E512 **Stannous Chloride Or Tin Chloride.** Reducing agent, Anti-oxidant, Color retention agent.	$SnCl_2$ Stannous chloride is made by dissolving tin in hydrochloric acid. Used in canned foods, such as canned beans or asparagus. Can be used to test for the presence of gold compounds because $SnCl_2$ turns bright purple in the presence of gold. Caution may cause nausea, headache and gastric upset, it may cause liver or kidney damage and reduce blood pressure. It is a possible skin and mucous membrane irritant. Listed for UK, NZ, AU, USA, EU and CAN.
E513 **Sulfuric acid.** Acidity Regulator.	H_2SO_4, It is a strong mineral acid made by the oxidation of sulfur dioxide in the presence of water. Its main use is in beer. Banned in Australia and others, it has teratogenic (birth defect) properties. Listed for UK, EU, USA

	and CAN. Not listed for AU and NZ.
E514 **Sodium sulfates.** Anti caking agent.	Na_2SO_4 It is the sodium salt of sulfuric acid. Made by the oxidation of sulfur dioxide in the presence of water. Used in beer, biscuits, chewing gum and confectionary etc. Caution for those with heart, kidney or liver problems, children should avoid. It may upset the body's water balance. Listed for UK, NZ, AU, EU, USA and CAN.
E515 **Potassium sulfate.** Anti caking agent, Acidity regulator, Salt substitute.	K_2SO_4 It is made by mixing potassium chloride with sulfuric acid. Used in beer and low salt products etc. Considered safe in normal usage, but may cause intestinal bleeding and other problems with excessive amounts. Caution, it is known to be toxic in excess, people with kidney or liver problems have extra caution. Listed for UK, AU, NZ, USA, EU and CAN.
E516 **Calcium sulfate.** Stabilizer, Bleaching agent, Calcium	$CaSO_4,$ It is naturally in gypsum and anhydrite, which may be extracted by mining. Bleaching agent for bread rolls, and flour. Used in cheese products, dried eggs, tinned tomatoes, and as a calcium supplement. I would consider caution with excessive usage of any

supplement. Buffer, Firming agent. Sequestrant (Ties up other chemicals).	non food based supplements. Long term (months to years to decades) excessive usage of any single mineral supplement may disrupt the body's mineral balance. Considered safe with proper usage. Listed for UK, NZ, AU, USA, EU and CAN.
E517 **Ammonium sulfate.** Stabilizer and buffer, Fertilizer in soils.	$(NH_4)_2SO_4$, It is made by reacting ammonia with sulfuric acid. Used in baked products and in water purification. Excess ammonia is toxic, but found naturally in the body as it is a product of protein catabolism and is safely removed by the by the liver. Normal blood ammonia levels range from 10-40 µmol/L. This increases to 10% with exposure to 25 ppm, but is not considered harmful. People with liver dysfunction may be at increased risk for ammonia toxicity. Early symptoms of ammonia toxicity related to decreasing liver function include inability to concentrate, sleepiness and being prone to irritability. Listed for UK, EU and USA and CAN. Not listed for AU and NZ.
E518 **Magnesium sulfate,** **(Epsom**	$MgSO_4$, It is made from magnesium salts and sulfuric acid. A common health treatment when this salt is put in warm bath water. Used as a brewing

salts). Firming agent, Supplement.	salt in beer production. Laxative, and has many uses for medical treatments such as a magnesium supplement. Caution for those with kidney problems, generally safe in moderate usage. Caution using any non plant based mineral supplements excessively, over time may damage kidneys other organs. Any single mineral supplement used in excess over a long time (months to years to decades) may disrupt the body's mineral balance. Not listed for UK and EU. Listed for NZ, AU, CAN and USA.
E519 **Copper sulfate** Supplement.	$CuSO_4$, It is made by treating copper metal or its oxides with sulfuric acid. Traces are naturally found in meat, cereals, and vegetables, it is used as supplementation in agriculture and livestock feed to increase growth rate. It can also be used in infant formula as a mineral supplement. Essential mineral for many body functions such as making blood and tissues, to fighting infections. If taken in pure concentrated form it is a poison, usually will evoke vomiting. Consider caution when taking any non plant based supplement excessively and long term. Those with kidney or liver problems should

	avoid. May be neurotoxin and have mutating properties. This is an essential mineral, but caution with using excessive amounts of the manmade type. Any single mineral supplement used in excess over a long time (months to years to decades) may disrupt the body's internal balance. Not listed for UK, EU and CAN. Listed for AU, NZ and USA.
E520 **Aluminum sulfate.** Firming agent and acidity regulator.	$Al_2(SO_4)_3$ It is made by dissolving aluminum hydroxide in sulfuric acid. Used to purify drinking water, and in waste water treatment plants. In beer, pickled vegetables and deodorant etc. Aluminum inhibits the uptake of B-vitamins. Caution, long term intake of aluminum may cause bad health effects, such as mineral imbalances, memory problems, kidney damage, senility and mouth ulcers etc. Limit or avoid, note-concentrations commonly used in products are so tiny they are considered safe by some. Listed for UK, EU, USA and CAN. Not listed for AU and NZ.
E521 **Aluminum sodium sulfate**	$NaAl(SO_4)_2 \cdot 12H_2O$, It is made from natural aluminum sulfate, which is produced by dissolving aluminum hydroxide in sulfuric acid. Used in flour, cheese

Firming agent and acidity regulator, Bleaching agent.	and confectionary etc. Aluminum inhibits the uptake of B-vitamins. Caution, long term intake of aluminum may cause bad health effects, such as mineral imbalances, memory problems, kidney damage, senility and mouth ulcers etc. Limit or avoid, note-concentrations commonly used in products are so low they are considered safe by some. Listed for UK, EU, USA and CAN. Not listed for AU and NZ.
E522 Aluminum potassium sulfate. Stabilizer, Acidity regulator.	$KAl(SO_4)_2$, It is made by reacting potassium sulfate with aluminum sulfate, and then dissolving aluminum hydroxide in sulfuric acid. Used in baked foods etc. Aluminum inhibits the uptake of B-vitamins. Caution, long term intake of Aluminum may cause bad health effects, such as mineral imbalances, memory problems, kidney damage, senility and mouth ulcers etc. Limit or avoid, note-concentrations commonly used in products are so low they are considered safe by some. Listed for UK, EU, USA and CAN. Not listed for AU and NZ.
E523 **Aluminum ammonium**	$(NH_4)Al(SO_4)_2$ It is made by reacting ammonium sulfate with aluminum sulfate. Used in industrial baking powder etc. In

sulfate. Stabilizer, Firming agent, Raising agent, Acidity regulator.	pickled vegetables, seaweeds, flour, starches and egg-based desserts. Aluminum inhibits the uptake of B-vitamins. Caution, long term intake of Aluminum may cause bad health effects, such as mineral imbalances, memory problems, kidney damage, senility and mouth ulcers etc. Limit or avoid, note-concentrations commonly used in products are so tiny they are considered safe by some in terms of aluminum content. Excess ammonia is toxic, but naturally in the body as it is a product of protein catabolism and is safely removed by the by the liver. Normal blood ammonia levels range from 10-40 μmol/L. This increases 10% with exposure to 25 ppm, but is not considered harmful. People with liver dysfunction may be at increased risk for ammonia toxicity. Early symptoms of ammonia toxicity related to decreasing liver function include inability to concentrate, sleepiness and being prone to irritability. Listed for UK, EU, USA and CAN. Not listed for AU and NZ.
E524 **Sodium hydroxide Also called**	NaHO , It is made commercially by electrolysis of sodium chloride. It is a strong base in PH. Used in cocoa products, drain cleaners (in

Lye or Caustic Soda. Acidity regulator. Strong base in terms of PH.	concentration), sour cream, edible fats and oils, jams and jellies, tinned vegetables and black olives. Alters protein content of food, mutagen and corrosive in concentration. Not listed for AU and NZ. Listed for UK, USA, EU and CAN.
E525 **Potassium hydroxide Also called Caustic Potash.** Acidity regulator. Strong base in terms of PH.	KOH, It is made by the electrolysis of potassium chloride. It is a strong base. Used in cheese products, cocoa products, jams, and black olives. Corrosive in concentration, caused tumors on skin of mice in testing. Can cause gastro intestinal upset. Ingestion of Potassium hydroxide in concentration can cause death. Not listed for NZ and AU. Listed for UK, EU, USA and CAN.
E526 **Calcium hydroxide, Also called Slaked Lime or Pickling Lime.** Acidity regulator. Strong base in terms of PH.	$Ca(OH)_2$,, It is made by mixing calcium oxide with water. Used in making beer, soap, glazing pretzels, dried fish, in infant formula as a mineral, cocoa products, sour cream, edible fats, oils, jam and canned vegetables. Considered safe in small quantities, however concentrated calcium hydroxide is toxic. Listed for UK, NZ, AU, EU, USA and CAN.

E527 **Ammonium hydroxide. Also called Ammonium water.** Acidity regulator. Strong base in terms of PH.	NH_4OH, It is a solution of ammonia in water. Used in cocoa and egg products. Excess ammonia is toxic, but found naturally in the body as it is a product of protein catabolism and is safely removed by the by the liver. Normal blood ammonia levels range from 10-40 µmol/L. This increases to 10% with exposure to 25 ppm, but not considered harmful. People with liver dysfunction may be at increased risk for ammonia toxicity. Early symptoms of ammonia toxicity related to decreasing liver function include inability to concentrate, sleepiness and being prone to irritability. Banned in Australia and others, best to limit or avoid. Listed for UK, EU, USA and CAN. Not listed for AU and NZ.
E528 **Magnesium hydroxide. Common name is Milk of Magnesia.** Acidity regulator. Strong base in	$Mg(OH)_2$, It is precipitated by the reaction between magnesium salts and sodium, potassium, or ammonium hydroxide. Used in cheese and canned goods to stabilize color in vegetables. Commonly in antacids and laxatives; it interferes with the absorption of folic acid and iron. Diarrhea caused by magnesium hydroxide carries away much of the body's potassium, and failure to take

terms of PH.	in extra potassium may lead to muscle cramps. Banned in Australia and others, best to avoid or limit usage. Listed for UK, EU and CAN. Not listed for AU and NZ.
E529 **Calcium oxide. Also called Quicklime or Burnt Lime.** Acidity regulator and Stabilizer.	CaO, It is made by heating limestone, coral, sea shell or chalk, all contain calcium carbonate-to cook off the carbon dioxide leaving the calcium oxide behind. Used in bread, cocoa, confectionary, sour cream, dairy products, tripe, canned peas and sausage casings. Considered safe in small quantities. Listed for UK, NZ, AU, EU, USA and CAN.
E530 **Magnesium oxide.** Acidity regulator, Anti caking agent, Supplement.	MgO, It is prepared from several mined minerals. Used in baked products, frozen dairy, canned peas, butter, and cocoa products. In antacids for heartburn and sore stomach, used as a magnesium supplement, and a short-term laxative. In medical usage, it is used to improve symptoms of indigestion. Side effects of magnesium oxide may include nausea and cramping—in quantities sufficient to obtain a laxative effect. Effect of excessive long-term use may be mineral concentrations or balls inside intestines resulting in

	bowel obstruction. Causes cancer in hamsters, can cause diarrhea. Banned in Australia and others, best to avoid, or limit usage. Listed for UK, NZ, AU, EU, USA and CAN.
E535 **Sodium ferrocyanide.** Anti caking agent.	$Na_4Fe(CN)_6$ Made when hydrogen ferrocyanide and sodium hydroxide are combined. Normally a yellow powder, but when combined with iron it converts to a deep blue pigment called Prussia blue. Rarely used because of it's yellow color. No known bad effects when used in food. Listed for UK, AU, NZ, EU, USA and CAN.
E536 **Potassium ferrocyanide.** Acidy regulator, Anti caking agent.	$C_6N_6FeK_4$ It is made when hydrogen ferrocyanide and potassium hydroxide are combined. A byproduct of coal gas production. An anti caking agent that can be used in herbal salts, table salt and road salt. Reduces oxygen transport in the blood, if sensitive it may cause breathing difficulties, dizziness and or headache, or if too much is ingested in non proper usage. Not listed for CAN. Listed for UK, NZ, AU, USA and EU.
E537 **Ferrous hexacyanom**	It is made by adding hydrogen manganocyanide and iron hydroxide together. Used in licorice powder (salmiak). No known side effects in

anganate. Anti caking agent.	proper concentrations commonly used. Not listed for UK, NZ, AU, EU, USA and CAN.
E538 **Calcium ferrocyanid e.** Anti caking agent.	Ca2Fe(CN)6·12H2O It is made from a combination of hydrogen ferrocyanide and calcium hydroxide. Used as a low-sodium salt substitute. Acceptable daily intake, up to 25 mg/kg of bodyweight. No known bad effects with acceptable daily intake. Caution with excessive usage. Listed for UK, USA and EU. Not listed for AU, NZ and CAN.
E539 **Sodium thiosulfate.** Anti Oxidant, Sequestrant (binding agent).	$Na_2S_2O_3$ It is made from the liquid waste products of sodium sulfide. It is an antidote to cyanide poisoning. Thiosulfate acts as a sulfur donor for the conversion of cyanide to thiocyanate. Use as an antioxidant which prevents browning in potato products etc. Thiosulfate is converted into sulfite, it has a similar effects as all sulfites, caution, see E220. Not listed for UK, AU, NZ and EU and CAN. Listed for USA.
E540 **Dicalcium diphosphate** Stabilizer,	$CaHPO_4 • 2H_2O$ Dicalcium phosphate can be formed by equal amounts (by the mole) of calcium carbonate and phosphoric acid. It is used in cupcake mixes, pie tops, instant pastas and sauces,

Acidity regulator, Sequestrant (binding agent), Emulsifier(mixing agent).	muesli bars, ice-cream, and instant soups. Used to retain water in processing and storage. Buffer, neutralizing and raising agent in yeast products, a dietary supplement. Not listed for UK, EU, NZ, AU, USA and CAN.
E541a **Sodium aluminum phosphate - acidic.** Acidity regulator, Emulsifier(mixing agent), Raising agent, Acid in PH.	NaAlPO4 It is made from aluminum, phosphoric acid and sodium hydroxide. Used in baked goods, dry prepared mixes such as cake and pancake mixes. Thought to release aluminum during digestion. Aluminum impairs calcium and phosphorous uptake by the body. Possible link to osteoporosis, Parkinson's and Alzheimer's disease. Banned in some countries. Listed for UK, AU, NZ, USA, EU and CAN.
E541b **Sodium aluminum phosphate - alkaline.** Acidity regulator, Emulsifier(mixing agent), Base in PH.	NaAlPO4 It is made from aluminum, phosphoric acid and sodium hydroxide. Used in baked goods, and processed cheese. Thought to release aluminum during digestion. Aluminum impairs calcium and phosphorous uptake by the body. Possible link to osteoporosis, Parkinson's and Alzheimer's disease. Banned in some countries. Listed for UK, NZ, AU, EU, USA and CAN.

E542 **Bone phosphate.** Anti caking agent, Emulsifier (mixing agent), Sequestrant (binding agent), Vitamin supplement.	PO4 It is made from animal bones. A source of phosphorous for food supplements. Used in dried coffee whiteners, cane sugar, and as filler in tablets, tooth paste and cosmetics. Generally considered safe, may be made of pig bones. Not listed for UK, USA, EU and CAN. Listed for AU and NZ.
E543 **Calcium sodium polyphosph ate.** Emulsifier (mixing agent), Raising agent, Sequestrant (binding agent), Stabilizer.	It is made from a mixture of calcium and sodium salts of polyphosphoric acids. Used in cheese and frozen baked goods etc. Polyphosphates may inhibit digestive enzymes in high concentrations. Acceptable daily intake, up to 70 mg/kg bodyweight. Not much information. Not listed for UK, EU, NZ, AU, USA and CAN.
E544 **Calcium**	A mixture of calcium salts of polyphosphoric acids. These salts are used for dairy and cheese products. It

polyphosph ates. Emulsifier (mixing agent), Sequestrant (binding agent).	may cause enzyme blocking in the digestive system and also a calcium phosphorous imbalance. Not listed for UK, NZ, AU, USA, CAN and EU.
E545 **Ammonium polyphosph ates.** Anti caking agent, Emulsifier (mixing agent), Sequestrant (binding agent).	$[NH_4 PO_3]_n$ It is made from an salt of polyphosphoric acid and ammonia. Used in cheese, frozen poultry, chewing gum, beer, processed nuts, confectionary, herbal teas, chewing gum, beer, cider, herb teas, confectionary and processed nuts. Also used as nutrient for yeast and to increases water binding properties. Excess ammonia is toxic, but found naturally inside the body because it is a product of protein catabolism and is safely removed by the liver. Normal blood ammonia levels range from 10-40 µmol/L. This increases to 10% with exposure to 25 ppm, but is not considered harmful. People with liver dysfunction may be at increased risk for ammonia toxicity. Early symptoms of ammonia toxicity related to decreasing liver function include inability to concentrate, sleepiness and being

	prone to irritability. Not listed for UK, USA, CAN, NZ, AU and EU.
E546 **Magnesium pyrophosph ate.** Anti caking agent, Emulsifier (mixing agent).	$Mg_2O_7P_2$ It is made when sodium phosphate is added to magnesium sulfate in the presence of ammonia and ammonium chloride, which is then heated to over 100 degrees. No known common usages, not much information. Not listed for UK, NZ, AU, USA and CAN.
E550 **Sodium silicate.** Buffer, Anti caking agent.	$Na_2 O_3 Si$ It is an inorganic compound that is made by combining various ratios of sand (silicon dioxide, quartz) with sodium carbonate (soda ash) at very high temperatures. It is soluble in water. Used in preserving eggs, vanilla powder, and canned peaches etc. No known bad effects. Not listed for UK, NZ, AU and EU. Listed for USA and CAN.
E551 **Silicon dioxide (Silica).** Vitamin supplement,	SiO_2 It is the most abundant mineral in the earth's crust. Commonly used in making glass. In foods used in beer, dried milk, confectionary, sausages, powdered sugars, processed cheese, fat spreads, and salt etc. Silica is very dangerous to breath and will cake up

Thickener, Stabilizer, Anti caking agent.	the lungs over time, avoid this. No known bad effects in foods. Listed for UK, EU, NZ, AU, USA and CAN.
E552 **Calcium silicate.** Anti caking agent, anti acid.	Ca_2SiO_4 It is made by reacting calcium oxide and silica in various ratios or made from limestone and diatomaceous earth (the silicified skeletons of diatoms, a single celled plankton). Used as an antacid, glaze, polishing, releasing, dusting agent in chewing gum and as a coating agent on rice. It is a powder that can absorb large amounts of water. No known bad effects. Listed for UK, NZ, AU, USA, EU and CAN.
E553a **Magnesium silicates,** **1.** **Magnesium silicate** **2.Magnesiu m trisilicate** **or** **Talcum Powder.** Anti caking agent, Dusting agent, Coating	$Mg_3Si_4O_{10}(OH)_2$ It is made by hydrating silicate salts of magnesium. Antacid, glazing agent, polishing agen, releasing agent, anti-caking agent, dusting agent and coating agent. Generally recognized as safe when used properly in small quantities. Can be damaging to breath the powder and some testing indicates that it can be related to cancer. (A 1971 paper found particles of talc embedded in 75% of the ovarian tumors studied.- Wikipedia) Be cautious of excessive daily usage. Listed for UK, NZ, AU, USA, EU and CAN.

agent.	
E553b **Talc** **or** **Talcum** **powder.** Anti caking agent.	$Mg_3Si_4O_{10}(OH)_2$ Made from magnesium sulfate and sodium silicate or directly from minerals such as talcum, sepiolite and steatite Typical products are polished rice, chocolate, confectionary, icing sugar, noodles, medicinal tablets and medications. Linked to stomach and ovarian cancers, may cause respiratory problems when breathed. A 1971 paper found particles of talc embedded in 75% of the ovarian tumors studied (Wikapedia). Talc dust may cause health problems over time (tumors), example, from cosmetic usage over a long period of time. Best to limit or avoid. Listed for UK, NZ, AU, USA, EU and CAN.
E554 **Sodium** **aluminum** **silicate.** Anti caking agent.	$AlNa_{12}SiO_5$ It is a mineral salt, a natural compound that contains silicon, sodium, aluminum, and oxygen. It can be made in a wide range of compositions to suit many different applications. Used in salt, dried milk substitutes, egg mixes, sugar products, and flours. Linked to Alzheimer's and nerve damage, bone diseases, kidney damage, and neurotoxicity. Aluminum may be linked to many health problems,

	including senility, neurological problems, mineral imbalances, mouth ulcers etc, best to avoid or limit. Listed for UK, NZ, AU, EU, USA and CAN.
E555 **Potassium aluminum silicate or Microcline.** Anti caking agent.	$KAlSi_3O_8$ It is a naturally occurring mineral found in rock. It is formed by aluminum silicate weakly bonded together by layers of potassium ions. Used in dry powdered mixes, but rarely used to date. No known bad effects, but caution due to aluminum content. Aluminum may be linked to many health problems, including senility, kidney problems, mineral imbalances and neurological problems etc. Listed for UK, AU, NZ and EU. Not listed for CAN and USA.
E556 **Calcium aluminum silicate. or Calcium aluminosilic ate** Anti caking agent.	$CaAl_2Si_2O_8$ Naturally occurring silicate clay, also can be produced from many natural minerals. Used in dry powdered mixes, but hardly used to date. Caution due to aluminum content. Aluminum may be linked to many health problems, including senility, kidney problems, mineral imbalances and neurological problems etc. Listed for UK, NZ, AU, EU, USA and CAN.
E557	$Zn_4Si_2O_7(OH)_2 \cdot H_2O$ Most frequently occurs as the

Zinc silicate or Hemimorphite. Anti caking agent.	product of the oxidation of the upper parts of sphalerite bearing ore bodies. Can be synthetically produced from quartz and zinc oxide. Used in dry products such as dry powders. Rarely used and is restricted. Not listed for EU, UK, NZ, AU, USA and CAN.
E558 **Bentonite.** Anti caking agent, Emulsifier (mixing agent).	$Al_2O_34SiO_2H_2O$ It is a natural clay from volcanic origin. There are different types of bentonite, each named after the respective dominant element, such as potassium (K), sodium (Na), calcium (Ca), and aluminum (Al). Used in pharmaceutical agents for external use, in edible fats, oils, sugar, wine, honey, beer and mineral water. Known to block skin pores, no known other bad effects. Listed for NZ, UK, AU, EU and USA. Not listed for CAN.
E559 **Aluminum silicate (Kaolin).** Anti caking agent.	Al_2SiO A clay mineral that is mined, treated for impurities, and then dried. Used in instant coffee, milk powder, aromas, antacid, medications and vending machine dried milk. Also used in cosmetics and blocks skin pores. No known bad health effects in food, except in large quantities can cause intestinal obstruction and tumors. Not listed for CAN and USA.

	Listed for UK, AU and NZ.
E560 **Potassium silicate.** Anti caking agent.	K_2O_3Si A naturally occurring compound that is the potassium salt of silica acid. It is water soluble. Potassium silicate is a natural active ingredient that is used as a fungicide, insecticide and miticide. Currently seldom used as food additive, not much information in use as a food additive. Not listed for USA, UK, EU and CAN. Listed for AU and NZ.
E570 **Stearic acid.** Anti caking agent, Glazing agent.	$C_{18}H_{36}O_2$ A natural saturated fatty acid, it is industrially made by treating animal fat with water at high temperature and pressure. Fat may be of pig origin. It can also be made by the hydrogenation of some vegetable oils. Also stearic acid is made by the mixture of stearic acid and palmitic acid. Used in chewing gum, butter flavors, baked products, dietary supplements, soft drinks, vanilla flavoring and artificial sweeteners. May cause allergic reactions in sensitive people and possible skin irritant. Listed for UK, AU, NZ, EU, USA and CAN.
E571 **Ammonium stearate.**	C18H39NO2 Ammonium salt of stearic acid is a natural saturated fatty acid used in sugar and bakery products. Excess

Anti caking agent, Anti foaming agent.	ammonia is toxic, but naturally found in the body as a product of protein catabolism and is safely removed by the by the liver. Normal blood ammonia levels range from 10-40 µmol/L. This increases 10% with exposure to 25 ppm, but is not considered harmful. People with liver dysfunction may be at increased risk for ammonia toxicity. Early symptoms of ammonia toxicity related to decreasing liver function include inability to concentrate, sleepiness and being prone to irritability. Caution see E570. Not listed for UK, AU, NZ, USA and CAN.
E572 **Magnesium stearate, Calcium stearate.** Anti caking agent, Emulsifier (mixing agent), Stabilizer, Releasing agent.	$Mg(C_{18}H_{35}O_2)_2$ and $C_{36}H_{70}CaO_4$ Magnesium stearate and calcium stearate are the magnesium and calcium salts of stearic acid. Used in capsules and tablets, baby formula, bakery products, artificial sweeteners, confectionary, and baby powders. No known bad effects in acceptable usage in food. Not listed for UK, NZ, AU and EU. Listed for USA and CAN.
E573	$C_{18}H_{37}AlO_4$ A natural saturated fatty acid, it is

Aluminum Stearate. Anti caking agent.	industrially made by treating animal fat with water at high temperature and pressure, source fat may be of pig origin. It can also be made by hydrogenation of some vegetable oils, may be genetically modified. Also stearic acid is made by the mixture of stearic acid and palmitic acid. Caution due to aluminum content, aluminum may be linked to many health problems, including senility, kidney problems, neurological problems, mineral imbalances and mouth ulcers etc. Not listed for UK, NZ, AU and CAN. Listed for USA.
E574 **Gluconic acid.** Acidy regulator.	$C_6H_{12}O_7$ It is a naturally occurring substance that is found in fruit, honey, tea and wine. It can also be made by the fermentation of glucose with certain moulds. It is a strong chelating agent, especially in an alkaline solution. It chelates the cations of calcium, iron, aluminum, copper, and other heavy metals. Used in cleaning products to remove alkali mineral deposits. Used in processed fruits and vegetables, soft drinks, desserts, milk products, and beer. Not much information on safety. Listed for UK, EU, USA and CAN. Not listed for AU and NZ.
E575	$C_6H_{10}O_6$

Glucono delta-lactone. Acidy regulator, Sequestrant(b inding agent), Leavening agent(causes fermentation), Artificial sweetener base.	A natural ester of gluconic acid, which is created by the fermentation of glucose. Found in gluten free food and processed meat. Used in sausage, canned fish and shellfish, processed vegetables, processed meat, cheese, and baking powder. No known bad effects. Listed for UK, EU, AU, NZ, USA and CAN.
E576 **Sodium gluconate.** Sequestrant(b inding agent), Stabilizer.	$C_6H_{11}NaO_7$ It is a sodium salt of gluconic acid, see E574. Found in fruit, honey, tea and wine. It can be made by the fermentation of glucose with certain molds. Picks up metal traces and holds them in the product. Dietary supplement, also found in baked goods, confectionary, soft, sports and fizzy drinks, processed meats and desserts. May be corn based, may be genetically modified, may cause kidney problems, high blood pressure and water retention. Allowed in UK, USA, EU and CAN. Not listed for AU, NZ and others.
E577	$C_6H_{11}KO_7$ Potassium salt of gluconic acid, that

Potassium gluconate. Anti oxidant, Squestrant(bi nding agent) Stabalizer, Mineral supplement.	is found in fruit, honey, tea and wine. It can be made by the fermentation of glucose with certain molds. A commonly used potassium supplement, also used in puddings powders and custards. No known bad effects, but caution excessively using non food based supplements. Listed for UK, EU, NZ, AU and USA. Not listed for CAN.
E578 **Calcium gluconate.** Firming agent, Buffer, Sequestrant(b inding agent), Acidity regulator, Artificial sweetener base, Mineral supplement.	$C_{12}H_{22}CaO_{14}$ Calcium salt of gluconic acid, that is found in fruit, honey, tea and wine. It can be made by the fermentation of glucose with certain molds. Used in dietary supplements, processed meats, table-top sweeteners, bakery goods, batters, breakfast cereals, and infant formula supplements. No known bad effects as food additive. Listed for UK, NZ, AU, EU, USA and CAN.
E579 **Ferrous gluconate.** Color agent(black), Iron	$C_{12}H_{24}FeO_{14}$ Iron salt of gluconic acid, which is a naturally occurring compound that is found in fruit, honey, tea, and wine. It can be made by the fermentation of glucose with certain molds. Used in olives, canned foods and iron supplements. Caution as little as 1-2

supplement.	grams can kill small children less than 24 months old. Acceptable daily intake is up to 0.8 mg/kg bodyweight. May cause gastrointestinal stress, considered generally safe in proper usage by industry, need more research. Caution in taking non food based supplements excessively long term. Listed for UK, EU, NZ, AU, USA and CAN.
E580 **Magnesium gluconate.** Acidity regulator, Firming agent, Yeast nutrient, Mineral supplement.	$C_{12}H_{22}MgO_{14}$ Magnesium salt of gluconic acid is found in fruit, honey, tea, and wine. It can be made by the fermentation of glucose with certain molds. Used in dietary supplements, milk powder and cream powder, processed cheese, fat spreads, processed fruits, canned or bottled vegetables, confectionary, and bakery products. Relatively new to date, not much information, caution. Not listed for UK, EU and CAN. Listed for NZ, AU and USA.
E585 **Ferrous lactate.** Acidity regulator, Color retention	$C_6H_{10}FeO_6$ Iron salt of lactic acid, which is a natural acid produced by the fermentation of milk sugar or lactose. It is made commercially from the bacterial fermentation of carbohydrates and molasses. Commercial ferrous lactate is not made from milk, so those with milk

agent.	allergy can use. Used as an iron supplement in foods and infant formulas. No known bad effects, may need more testing. Listed for UK, EU and USA. Not listed for NZ, AU and CAN.
E586 **4-Hexylresorcinol.** Anti-browning agent, Anti-oxidant agent, Color retention agent.	$C_{12}H_{18}O_2$ Anaesthetic, antiseptic and antihelmintic(expels parasites) properties. It can be used topically on small skin infections, or as an ingredient in throat lozenges-used in antiseptic drops. A study published in Chemical Research in Toxicology in March 2009 shows that 4-hexylresorcinol used as a food additive (E-586) exhibits some estrogenic activity, i.e. resembles action of the female sex hormone estrogen. Not much information, caution. Not listed for UK, EU and USA. Listed for NZ, AU and CAN.
E598 **Synthetic calcium aluminates.** Binder, Anti-caking agent.	Created by burning high grade crude aluminous bauxite and limestone in an arc-furnace kiln. Currently to date only used in animal feed. Aluminum can be toxic in at a too great concentration. Aluminum may be linked to many health problems, including senility, kidney problems, neurological problems and mineral imbalances etc. Not listed for UK, NZ, AU, USA, EU and CAN.

E599 **Perlite.** Bulking agent, Filtering agent.	A siliceous rock formed by volcanic action, which is mined and then ground into a coarse to fine white powder. Can expand 7 to 16 times its size when heated. It is mainly used to filter liquids and does not alter taste or color of liquids it filters. In the construction and manufacturing fields, it is used in lightweight plasters and mortars, insulations and ceiling tiles. Not listed for UK, USA, NZ, AU, EU and CAN.

Flavors & Flavor Enhancers E620-E640:

Flavor additives are given to food for a particular taste or smell, and may be derived from natural ingredients or created artificially.

Flavor enhancers, (such as monosodium glutamate or MSG), enhance food's existing flavor. They are often added to commercially produced food, for example-frozen dinners, instant soups, and snack foods to make them tastier.

E620 **Glutamic acid.** Flavor enhancer, Salt substitute, Dietary supplement	$C_5H_9NO_4$ Commercially made from molasses by bacterial fermentation, also made from vegetable protein (Source vegetable may be genetically modified soy etc). Flavor enhancer, and salt substitute used in sausages, seasoning, savory snacks processed cheese, fat spreads, seasonings, condiments, soups and broths, in

many savory foods. Glutamic acid is a non essential acid, but still is very important for body function and is found naturally in many plants and foods. It is a major component for creating good taste in foods with protein. Considered to create similar health problems as MSG see E621. May cause allergic or adverse reactions in sensitive people, children should avoid. May cause or aggravate diseases that are from nerve damage such as Huntington's, Alzheimer's and Parkinson's. Symptoms include headaches, nausea, sleeplessness, may cause very slight reaction so must pay close attention to all foods eaten to determine cause and effect. Understand that any adverse food reaction can have many different causes and it may be difficult to determine the cause, as often foods are in mixtures of fats, proteins and other additives. If you suspect a acute allergic reaction to MSG, you may want to investigate to make certain, also consider seeing a physician for allergy testing. To truly avoid additives you must reduced processed foods close to zero in diet. Remember additives lower than one percent may be legally not on label.

	Listed for UK, NZ, AU, EU and USA. Not listed for CAN.
E621 **Monosodiu m L-glutamate or MSG.** Flavor enhancer, Salt substitute.	$C_5H_8NNaO_4$ Monosodium Glutamate, commonly known as MSG, is a sodium salt of the amino acid (L-glutamic acid). It is a white crystalline substance soluble in water and alcohol. It is practically odorless. MSG is used to intensify flavors of foods. It is produced by a bacterial fermentation process with starch or molasses as carbon sources and ammonium salts as nitrogen sources. MSG is not a direct taste enhancer, but a flavor enhancer for gravies, meats, poultry, sauces, and in other combinations, Used in sausages, seasoning, savory snacks processed cheese, fat spreads, seasonings and condiments, soups and broths, in many savory foods. Traditionally known in alternative health sources as unhealthy, but at the same time, there are scientific studies that show acute negative effect is non existent for most people. I would err on the side of caution as long term negative effect may happen without noticeable short term bad reactions. It is noted that a certain percentage of the population - less than one percent have an acute reaction to MSG, resource in

Wikipedia.
http://en.wikipedia.org/wiki/Monos
odium_glutamate

MSG is in many, many foods sometimes under names that hide its content because it is a well known unpopular food additive. The term "natural flavor" is now often used by the food industry when using glutamic acid (MSG without the sodium salt attached). It may cause allergic reactions for sensitive people, children should avoid. May cause or aggravate diseases due to nerve damage such as Huntington's, Alzheimer's and Parkinson's. Symptoms of acute allergy include headaches, nausea, sleeplessness. It may cause slight reaction so must pay close attention to determine cause and effect. It may be hidden in many foods including infant formulas. It may increase appetite and cause a kind of food addiction. Remember that any adverse food reaction can have many different causes and it may be difficult to determine the cause, as foods are mixtures of fats, proteins and other additives. To avoid additives you must reduced all processed foods close to zero. Additives less than one percent may not be on the food label.

	Listed for UK, NZ, AU, EU and USA. Not listed for CAN.
E622 **Monopotass ium L-glutamate.** Flavor enhancer, Salt substitute.	$C_5H_8KNO_4$ It is the potassium acid salt of glutamic acid, see E620. Commercially glutamate is made by yeast or bacterial fermentation of molasses, starch, sugar beets, or sugar cane, or soy, or gluten (any of these may be genetically modified). Flavor enhancer, salt substitute used in sausages, seasoning, savory snacks processed cheese, fat spreads, seasonings and condiments, soups and broths. It is in many savory foods. Caution for people with poor kidney function, some symptoms are kidney pain, headache, asthma, nausea, restlessness, vomiting, diarrhea, and abdominal cramps. Extra caution for those with impaired kidneys or for infants, see E621. Listed for UK, NZ, AU, EU and USA. Not listed for CAN.
E623 **Calcium diglutamate** . Flavor enhancer, Salt substitute.	$C_{10}H_{16}CaN_2O_8$ It is the calcium acid salt of glutamic acid, it's the calcium analog of monosodium glutamate (MSG). Commercially glutamate is made by yeast or bacterial fermentation of molasses, starch, sugar beets, or sugar cane, or soy, or gluten (any of these may be genetically modified). It

	is a flavor enhancer, salt substitute used in sausages, seasoning, savory snacks processed cheese, fat spreads, seasonings and condiments, soups and broths, in many savory foods. Because the glutamate is the actual flavor-enhancer, it has the same flavor-enhancing properties as MSG, but without the increased sodium content. Asthmatics and aspirin sensitive people should avoid as they may have acute reaction. See E621. Listed for UK, EU, AU, NZ and USA. Not listed for CAN.
E624 **Monoammo nium L-glutamate.** Flavor enhancer, Salt substitute.	$C_5H_{12}N_2O_4$ The ammonium acid salt of glutamic acid, commercially glutamate is made by yeast or bacterial fermentation of molasses, starch, sugar beets, or sugar cane, or soy, or gluten (any of these may be genetically modified). It is a flavor enhancer, salt substitute used in sausages, seasoning, savory snacks processed cheese, fat spreads, seasonings and condiments, soups and broths, in many savory foods. Generally no acute reactions for most people, but asthmatics should avoid and potential for adverse reaction for sensitive people. Excess ammonia is toxic, but naturally found in the body as it is a product of protein

	catabolism and is safely removed by the by the liver. Normal blood ammonia levels range from 10-40 µmol/L. This increases 10% with exposure to 25 ppm, but is not considered harmful. People with liver dysfunction may be at increased risk for ammonia toxicity. Early symptoms of ammonia toxicity related to decreasing liver function include inability to concentrate, sleepiness and being prone to irritability. Listed for UK, NZ, AU, EU and USA. Not listed for CAN.
E625 **Magnesium diglutamate** . Flavor enhancer, Salt substitute.	$C_{10}H_{16}MgN_2O_8$ The magnesium acid salt of glutamic acid, commercially glutamate is made by yeast or bacterial fermentation of molasses, starch, sugar beets, or sugar cane, or soy, or gluten (any of these may be genetically modified). It is a flavor enhancer and salt substitute, can be in any savory food but rarely used and usually only in low sodium meat products. Generally no acute reactions for most people, but asthmatics should avoid and a potential for adverse reaction in sensitive people. Listed for UK, AU, NZ, EU. Not listed for CAN and USA.
E626	$C_{10}H_{14}N_5O_8P$ Guanylic acid is a natural acid, which

219

Guanylic acid or **5'-guanidylic acid or (GMP).** Flavor enhancer.	is part of RNA. It is one of the genetic carrier molecules in the cell and is in all living cells. Made from yeast extract, or from dried fish (sardines) or from seaweed. Used in sausages, seasoning, savory snacks processed cheese, fat spreads, seasonings, condiments, soups and broths, in many savory foods. Asthmatic people should avoid guanylic acid and guanylates. Because guanylates are metabolized to purines, they should be avoided by people suffering from gout. Listed for UK and EU. Not listed for AU, NZ, USA and CAN.
E627 **Disodium guanylate or Sodium 5'-guanylate or Disodium 5'-guanylate.** Flavor enhancer.	$C_{10}H_{12}N_5Na_2O_8P$ The disodium salt of guanylic acid also known as GMP, commercially it is made from dried fish, or yeast extract, or dried seaweed. It is a fairly expensive additive so it is usually not used independently of glutamic acid or monosodium glutamate (MSG), see E621. May be used in instant noodles, potato chips and snacks, tinned vegetables, cured meats, packet soup, in any processed savory food item. Disodium guanylate is not safe for babies under twelve weeks, and should generally be avoided by asthmatics and people with gout, because guanylates are metabolized to purines. But, the typical amounts

219

	found in food are usually too low to produce significant notable side effects for most people, unless eaten excessively over a period of time-months to years. It is hard to feel ongoing slight negative effects if present. Asthmatics and aspirin sensitive people should avoid, linked to hyperactivity for children, gout sufferers should avoid. Prohibited in foods for infants and young children. Listed for UK, AU, NZ, USA and EU. Not listed for CAN.
E628 **Dipotassiu m guanylate.** Flavor enhancer.	$C_{10}H_{12}K_2N_5O_8P$ It is a potassium salt of guanylic acid, commercially it is made from dried fish, oryeast extract, or dried seaweed. May be used in instant noodles, potato chips and snacks, tinned vegetables, cured meats, packet soup, in any processed savory food item. It is not safe for babies under twelve weeks, and should be avoided by asthmatics and people with gout, as guanylates are metabolized to purines. But, the typical amounts found in food are usually too low to produce significant notable side effects in most people, unless eaten excessively over a period of time-months to years. Hard to determine slight negative effects if present. Asthmatics and aspirin

	sensitive people should avoid, linked to hyperactivity for children, gout sufferers should avoid. Prohibited in foods for infants and young children. Listed for UK and EU. Not listed for AU, NZ, USA and CAN.
E629 **Calcium guanylate.** Flavor enhancer.	$C_{10}H_{12}CaN_5O_8P$ The calcium salt of guanylic acid, commercially it is made from dried fish, yeast extract or dried seaweed. Used in low salt or low sodium products, may be used in instant noodles, potato chips, snacks, tinned vegetables, cured meats, packet soup, in any processed savory food item. It is not safe for babies under twelve weeks, should be avoided by asthmatics and people with gout, as guanylates are metabolized to purines. However, typical amounts found in food are usually too low to produce significant side effects in most people, unless eaten excessively over a period of time-months to years. It is hard to determine slight negative effects if present. Asthmatics and aspirin sensitive people should avoid, linked to hyperactivity for children, gout sufferers should avoid. Prohibited in foods for infants and young children. Listed for UK and EU. Not listed for AU, NZ, CAN and USA.

E630 **Inosinic acid or IMP.** Flavor enhancer.	$C_{10}H_{13}N_4O_8P$ A natural acid that is mainly present in animals, commercially prepared from meat or fish (sardines). Also may be produced by bacterial fermentation of sugars (which may be from genetically modified plant sources). Used in fat spreads, fat-based desserts, processed fruit, dried vegetables, canned vegetables, breakfast cereals, pre-cooked pastas, batters, processed meat and poultry, fish products, processed cheese, egg-based desserts, seasonings and condiments, soups and broths. Used by athletes to increase the oxygen capacity of their blood. Inosinate can be manufactured into various compounds with the aid of genetically modified organisms: disodium inosinate E 631, dipotassium inosinate E 632, and dicalcium inosinate E 633. Inosinates may not be used in products intended for children under 12 weeks. Asthmatic people should avoid inosinates. Since inosinates are metabolised to purines, they should be avoided by people suffering from gout. Listed for UK and EU. Not listed for NZ, AU, CAN and USA.
E631	$C_{10}H_{11}N_4Na_2O_8P$ The disodium salt of inosinic acid,

Disodium inosinate. Flavor enhancer.	generally made from meat or from fish, or it may be produced from tapioca starch without any animal products. Used in fat spreads, fat-based desserts, processed fruit, dried vegetables, canned vegetables, breakfast cereals, pre-cooked pastas, batters, processed meat and poultry, fish products, processed cheese, egg-based desserts, seasonings and condiments, soups and broths. Since inosinates are metabolized to purines, they should be avoided by people suffering from gout. It may trigger gout symptoms, varied reactions reported, prohibited in foods for infants and young children. Not recommended for asthmatics. Listed for UK, AU, NZ, USA and EU. Not listed for CAN.
E632 **Dipotassiu m inosinate** Flavor enhancer.	$C_{10}H_{13}N_4O_8P.2K$ The potassium salt of inosinic acid is commercially prepared from meat or fish (sardines), may be produced by bacterial fermentation of sugars (which may be from genetically modified plant sources). Mainly used in low salt or low sodium products, used in fat spreads, fat-based desserts, processed fruit, dried vegetables, canned vegetables, breakfast cereals, pre-cooked pastas, batters, processed meat and poultry,

	fish products, processed cheese, egg-based desserts, seasonings and condiments, soups and broths. Since inosinates are metabolized to purines, they should be avoided by people suffering from gout. May trigger gout symptoms, varied reactions reported, prohibited in foods for infants and young children, not recommended for asthmatics. Listed for UK and EU. Not listed for AU, NZ, CAN and USA.
E633 **Calcium inosinate.** Flavor enhancer.	$C_{10}H_{11}CaN_4O_8P$ (xH_2O) The calcium salt of inosinic acid is commercially prepared from meat or fish (sardines), may be produced by bacterial fermentation of sugars (which may be from genetically modified plant sources). Mainly used in low salt or low sodium products, such as fat spreads, fat-based desserts, processed fruit, dried vegetables, canned vegetables, breakfast cereals, pre-cooked pastas, batters, processed meat and poultry, fish products, processed cheese, egg-based desserts, seasonings and condiments, soups and broths. Since inosinates are metabolized to purines, they should be avoided by people suffering from gout. May trigger gout symptoms, varied reactions reported, prohibited in

	foods for infants and young children. Not recommended for asthmatics. Listed for UK and EU. Not listed for AU, NZ, CAN and USA.
E634 **Calcium 5'-ribonucleotides.** Flavor enhancer.	$C_{10} H_{11} Ca N_4 O_8 P$ It is a mixture of calcium salts of guanylic (E626) and inosinic acid (E630). Mainly used in low salt or low sodium products, such as fat spreads, fat-based desserts, processed fruit, dried vegetables, canned vegetables, breakfast cereals, pre-cooked pastas, batters, processed meat and poultry, fish products, processed cheese, egg-based desserts, seasonings and condiments, soups and broths. Guanylates and inosinates, may not be used in products intended for children under 12 weeks. Asthmatic people should avoid guanylates and inosinates, as they are metabolised to purines, they should be avoided by people suffering from gout. However, concentrations used are generally so low that no acute effects are to be expected with moderate short term usage. Be careful of excessive ingestion over long periods of time (months to years to decades). Listed for UK and EU. Not listed for AU, NZ, CAN and USA.

E635	$C_{10}H_{11}N_4Na_2O_8P$
Disodium 5'-ribonucleotide. Flavor enhancer.	Made by mixing sodium salts of guanylic acid (E627) and disodium inosinate (E631). Used in fat spreads, fat-based desserts, processed fruit, dried vegetables, canned vegetables, breakfast cereals, pre-cooked pastas, batters, processed meat and poultry, fish products, processed cheese, egg-based desserts, seasonings, condiments, soups and broths. A mixture of 98% monosodium glutamate and 2% E635 has four times the flavor enhancing power of monosodium glutamate (MSG) alone. See E621. Check imported foods. May be associated with itchy skin rashes up to 30 hours after ingestion; rashes may vary from mild to dramatic; the reaction is dose-related and cumulative, for sensitive people; typical foods include flavored chips, instant noodles and party pies. Can cause terrible itchy skin rashes, hyperactivity, sleeplessness, mood changes, many varied ill effects reported. Avoid it-especially gout sufferers, asthmatics and aspirin sensitive people. Concentrations are so low that acute reaction is not expected for the majority of people. Listed for UK, AU, NZ and EU. Not listed for USA and CAN.

E636 **Maltol.** Flavor enhancer.	$C_6H_6O_3$ It is found in the bark of the larch tree, in pine needles, and in roasted malt (from which it gets its name), it may be produced synthetically by heating lactose and maltose. Because it has the odor of cotton candy and caramel, maltol is used to impart a sweet aroma to fragrances. Maltol's sweetness adds to the odor of freshly baked bread. Used in breads and cakes, sodas, ice creams, jam and chocolate substitutes etc. In large quantities it can help aluminum pass into the brain to cause Alzheimer's disease. Some countries ban its use for small children. Acceptable daily intake in sources: Up to 2 mg/kg of bodyweight. Not listed for UK, EU and CAN. Listed for AU, NZ and USA.
E637 **Ethyl maltol.** Flavor enhancer.	$C_7H_8O_3$ It is made from maltol (E636) by replacing one metholy group with an ethyl group. Used in dairy-based drinks, dairy-based desserts, chocolate products, chocolate substitutes, confectionary, chewing gum, baked goods, sports drinks, coffee, coffee substitutes, tea and wine products etc. It has a distinct caramel/butterscotch smell. Synthetically made, some concerns

	about toxicity, some countries ban it for small children. More study needed, caution. Not listed for UK, EU and CAN. Listed for AU, NZ and USA.
E640 **Glycine (and its sodium salts) or Glycol or Amino acetic acid.** Flavor enhancer.	$C_2H_5NO_2$ Glycine is a natural amino acid, a building block of protein, made from gelatin and partly synthetic. It is a nutrient, mainly for yeast in bread, used in pills, protein drinks, dietary supplements, antacids, analgesics, cough syrups, also a bread enhancer and as a sweetener. Other markets for USP grade glycine include its use as an additive in pet food and animal feed. For humans, glycine is sold as a sweetener/taste enhancer. Used in food, in supplements, and protein drinks. Certain drug formulations include glycine to improve gastric absorption of the drug. No known adverse affects in sources. Listed for UK, AU, NZ and EU and USA. Not listed for CAN.
E641 **Leucine.** Flavor	$C_6H_{13}NO_2$ It is synthesized from pyruvic acid by a series of enzymes. As an essential amino acid leucine is unable to be synthesized by animals, so it must be ingested. Leucine is the only dietary amino acid that has the capacity to stimulate muscle protein synthesis.

enhancer, Supplement.	All supplements of L-leucine should be balanced with supplements of L-isoleucine and L-valine at the same time. Supplementation must also be done in moderation as excess amounts can induce physical symptoms akin to hypoglycemia (low blood sugar). High levels of leucine supplements may also lead to disorders such as pellagra, which is chronic lack of niacin (vitamin B3) in the diet. High levels may also increase the total amount of ammonia found in the body of a person, so can be toxic. In general, supplementation of any kind should be done carefully, and not for long periods of time. Especially in excess, as imbalances may occur and sometimes supplements have impurities from manufacturing that can be harmful. Caution if you have kidney or liver impairment. Caution with kidneys if using in excess over a long period of time, it may damage kidneys. Not listed in UK and EU. Listed for AU, NZ, CAN and USA.
E642 **Lysine hydrochlori**	$C_6H_{14}N_2O_2$ L-lysine is usually manufactured by a fermentation process using Corynebacterium glutamicum; production exceeds 600,000 tons a year. As an essential amino acid it is

de or **Lysine.** Flavor enhancer, Supplement.	unable to be synthesized by animals so must be ingested. Lysine is an important additive to animal feed because it is a limiting amino acid. A common use is to try to suppress herpes. Most often made from soy, which may be genetically modified, so caution if have a soy allergy. If used in excess it will increase calcium uptake and create imbalances in the body's proteins. In general supplementation of any kind should be done carefully, and often not for long periods of time. Especially in excess, as imbalances may occur and sometimes supplements have impurities from manufacturing that can be harmful. Caution if have kidney or liver impairment, especially if using in excess over a long period of time. Not listed in UK, AU, NZ, EU and CAN. Listed for USA.
E650 **Zinc acetate.** Flavor enhancer, Supplement.	$C_4H_{10}O_6Zn$ Zinc acetates are prepared by the action of acetic acid on zinc carbonate or zinc metal. Used in lozenges, breath freshener, dietary supplements, chewing gum, body building formulas and supplements. Caution with using non plant based supplements in excess over a long period of time, as may be hard on

	organs and kidneys or cause imbalances. Listed for UK, USA and EU. Not listed for AU, NZ and CAN.
E700 to E799, Antibiotics	
E710 **Spiramycin.** Antibiotic, Anti-fungal, Anti-bacteria, Anti- parasite.	Spiramycin is widely used as a veterinary broad spectrum antibiotic for livestock, and residues can be found in meat, liver, kidney, milk and eggs. Used in EU, Canada and Mexico for treatment of the parasite Toxoplasmosis, it is not used in the USA. Many house cats carry this parasite and it can be transferred to humans by ingesting of feces from cats, or ingesting the infected meat of animals. Cats are a source of parasite infection to human hosts, although contact with raw meat, especially pork, is a more significant source in some countries. Fecal contamination of hands is a significant risk factor. People who own cats/animals should wash hands after petting, also when handling raw meat wash hands, do not eat undercooked meat. Consider a parasite cleanse program on a regular basis. It is estimated about half the world's human population has this parasite infection which usually is without symptoms, unless the immune system is weakened. (About 10%-30% of USA population is thought to have this parasite)

	Usually this parasite causes flu like symptoms for awhile and then obvious symptoms go away. The parasite can do damage to heart, liver, eyes (blindness) and brain during an acute infection which may happen later on in life. Latent infection without obvious symptoms can last for many years and even may cause behavior changes such as a more risk taking attitude, also skin rash, fatigue, muscle and joint pain, pneumonia, and central nervous system problems. A blood test can be done to determine infection. Spiramycin is used as an alternative agent in the treatment of toxoplasmosis during pregnancy. Side effects can happen when using spiramycin as antibiotic, not much information on safety as an item in food, may be a source of adverse reactions, caution. Not listed for UK, AU, NZ, USA, EU and CAN.
E713 **Tylosin** Antibiotic, Anti-fungal, Anti-bacteria.	C46H77NO17 Tylosin is a macrolide-class antibiotic used in veterinary medicine. It is used in veterinary medicine to treat bacterial infections in a wide range of species. Used as growth promotant in food producing animals. Tylosin is available in injectable, intramammary, and oral

	formulations, with different product ranges available in different countries. Found in dairy, meat, egg-products, only allowed with special permission. Acceptable daily intake, up to 0.2 mg/kg of bodyweight. Not much information on safety or possible adverse reactions, antibiotic bacteria should be killed by cooking if any still in animal during slaughter, (they are not take any antibiotics several days before slaughter), caution. Not listed for UK, NZ, AU, EU, USA and CAN.

Sweeteners, Humectants (water holding) or Antifoaming or Bulking Agents (and miscellaneous agents): E900 to E1520

Sweeteners are added to food to make them sweet. Sugar is most common or corn syrup, but there are others that make things sweet that are useful for diabetes suffers. Humectants help food to stay moist.

Antifoaming agents are used in production to reduce or prevent foaming in foods. Bulking agents such as starch are additives that increase the bulk of a food, to make it go farther or to improve body without affecting its nutritional value.

E900 **Polydimeth ylsiloxane**	$(C_2H_6OSi)_n$ A synthetically made silicone based oil, officially considered to be inert, non-toxic and non-flammable. Used in dairy products, chewing gum,

or **Dimethylpol ysiloxane.** Anti-foaming agent, Anti-caking agent.	vinegar, soups, jellies, beer, powdered milk, imitation chocolate, sports drinks, etc. May be cancer causing, may be contaminated with asbestos or formaldehyde, may cause kidney problems. Acute adverse reactions are not common, but consider limited intake. Listed for UK, AU, NZ, EU, USA and CAN.
E901 **Beeswaxes, white & yellow.** Glazing agent.	$C_{15}H_{31}COOC_{30}H_{61}$ A natural wax made by bees to make honeycomb that supports their honey and makes up their home. It is estimated that bees fly 150,000 miles, roughly six times around the earth, to yield one pound of beeswax. Used to wax fruit, confectionary, chocolate, ice cream, snack food coating for cheese, natural cosmetics, and food supplements. etc. White beeswax has been bleached, and yellow has not. May cause adverse reactions for sensitive people when used in cosmetics and foods. Listed for UK, AU, NZ, EU and USA. Not listed for CAN.
E902 **Candelilla wax.** Glazing agent.	Made from the leaves of the small Candelilla shrub native to northern Mexico and the southwestern United States. The wax is made by boiling the leaves and stems with dilute sulfuric acid, and the resulting "cerote" is skimmed from the surface

	and further processed. About 900 tons are produced annually. A glazing agent used to wax fruit and vegetables. It's cheaper than other waxes like Carnauba (E903) and paraffin so it is used as a substitute. Needs more research, no adverse reactions in sources. Listed for UK, EU, USA and CAN. Not listed for AU and NZ.
E903 **Carnauba wax** **or** **Brazil wax or Palm wax.** Glazing agent, Anti-caking agent.	It is known as the "queen of waxes", made from the leaves of the carnauba palm by collecting them, beating them to loosen the wax, then refining and bleaching the wax. It is a hard yellow-brown wax. Used in baked goods, chewing gum, cocoa, chocolate, coffee, frostings, to wax fruit and vegetables, and in sports drinks. It may cause allergic reactions on the skin in sensitive people, and is a possible cancer causing agent. Listed for UK, AU, NZ, USA, EU and CAN.
E904 **Shellac.** Glazing agent.	It is a natural, organic resin that is secreted by the female lac beetle on trees found in India and Thailand. It can be dissolved in ethyl alcohol to make liquid shellac, it is used as a brush-on colorant, food glaze and wood finish. Shellac also functions as a tough natural primer, sanding

	sealant, tannin-blocker, odor-blocker, stain, and high-gloss varnish. Used to make a shiny hard coating on candies and fruits, such as apples. It may cause adverse skin reactions. Listed for UK, EU, AU, NZ, USA and CAN.
E905 **Paraffins or** **Parraffin wax.** Glazing agent.	C_nH_{2n+2} Paraffin wax refers to a mixture of alkanes that falls within the $20 \leq n \leq 40$ range, they are found in the solid state at room temperature and begin to enter the liquid phase past approximately 37 °C (99 °F). Used as protective coating on fruit and also used as a glazing agent to give chocolate and confectionary a nice glossy finish. May cause adverse reactions, birth defects and cancer. Listed for USA, EU and CAN. Not listed for UK, AU and NZ.
E905a **Mineral oil.** Glazing agent, Non sticking agent used on baking pans.	Most often mineral oil is a liquid by-product of the distillation of petroleum in producing gasoline and other petroleum-based products from crude oil. A mineral oil in this sense is a transparent, colorless oil. Used as a chewing gum ingredient, sealant, glazing agent, de-foamer, food processing machine lubricant, protective coating on fruit, lubricant and binder for tablets and capsules. It may be related to bowel cancer and

	birth or developmental defects in children. Not listed for UK, NZ, AU and EU. Listed for CAN and USA.
E905b **Petrolatum (petroleum jelly),** **(Vaseline).** Medication, Moisturizer.	Petroleum jelly's effectiveness in accelerating wound healing stems from its sealing effect on cuts and burns, which inhibits germs from getting into the wound and keeps the injured area supple by preventing the skin's moisture from evaporating. Most petroleum jelly today is consumed as an ingredient in skin lotions and cosmetics. It can be used for fire starting tinder by lightly coating it on a cotton ball. Petroleum jelly should not be applied to the inside of the nose due to the risk of lipid pneumonia, due to the jelly going into the lungs. Petroleum jelly weakens latex condoms, increasing the chance of rupture. Rarely used as a food additive, when so it may block the absorption of fats. Sensitive people may have an adverse skin reaction to petroleum jelly. Not listed for UK and EU. Listed for AU, NZ, USA and CAN.
905 E c **Microcystall**	It is made by de-oiling petrolatum, as part of the petroleum refining process. Glazing agent used to wax fruit and vegetables or candy, in processing yeast, vitamin tablets, dried fruit, confectionary and

ine wax. Glazing agent.	collagen. It is a synthetic mixture of hydrocarbons, that may inhibit absorption of fats and fat soluble vitamins, a mild laxative, there may be a link to bowel cancer. Not listed for NZ, AU, USA, EU and CAN. Listed for UK.
E906 **Gum benzoic** **or** **Benzoin resin** **or** **Styrax resin** **or** **Gum Benjamin.** Glazing agent, Flavor enhancer.	It is a resin polymer derived from the bark of trees from the genus Styrax from Southeast Asia. Its principal component is benzoic acid. Formerly used as preservative in fats. At present mostly used as part of many flavors and essences. Found in many different products, but mainly in pharmaceuticals and perfumes, make up and incense. This weak acid and its salts are used as a food preservative in some countries by inhibiting the growth of mold, yeasts and some bacteria. It can be used in many kinds of drinks and foods. No adverse reactions listed in sources. Not listed for AU, UK, NZ and EU. Listed for USA and CAN.
E907 **Refined microcrysta**	Microcrystalline wax is a type of creamy white to dark brown wax produced by de-oiling of petrolatum as part of the petroleum refining process. Used to wax fruits and vegetables and candies and more. It

lline wax. Glazing agent.	is a synthetically made product from petroleum, banned in many countries, best to avoid. Need more testing. Not listed for UK, AU, NZ and CAN and USA.
E908 **Rice bran wax.** Glazing agent.	Rice bran wax is used in paper coating, textiles, explosives, fruit & vegetable coatings, pharmaceuticals, candles, waterproofing, printing inks, lubricants, crayons and adhesive. It may also serve as a substitute for Carnauba wax (E903). Not listed for UK, AU, NZ, EU and CAN. Listed for USA.
E909 **Spermaceti wax.** Glazing agents.	$C_{15}H_{31}COO-C_{16}H_{33}$. It is a wax present in the head cavities of the sperm whale. Spermaceti is created in the spermaceti organ inside the whale's head and connected to its nasal passage. Its biological function is uncertain, may be used to alter buoyancy. A large whale could have as much as 500 gallons. After international regulations concerning whaling, it is rarely harvested and sold. It is now replaced by synthetic spermaceti. Not listed for UK, AU, NZ, USA and EU. Listed for in CAN.
E910	$C_3H_7NO_2S$ It is a non-essential amino acid, which means that it is biosynthesized

L-cysteine. Glazing agent, Flour treatment agent, Flavor agent.	inside humans. It is found naturally in many foods such as egg yolks, meat and in many vegetables. The majority of L-Cysteine was once obtained industrially by hydrolysis of human hair, but in recent years 80% is produced from duck feathers, it also can be produced synthetically. The reaction of cysteine with sugars yields a meaty flavor to be used in cubed stock flavorings. It is also used as a processing aid for baking. Diabetics should know there are some reports that it may interfere with insulin. Also it may interact with monosodium glutamate (E621) in people who react to MSG, causing a set of adverse symptoms, including headache, burning sensations, dizziness and disorientation. Not listed for UK, AU, NZ, USA and EU. Listed for CAN.
E911 **Methyl esters of fatty acids.** Glazing agent.	It is a type of fatty acid ester (fat with alcohol) than can be produced by an alkali-catalyzed reaction between fats or fatty acids and methanol. It can be used as a flavoring agent and glazing agent. No information on safety from listed sources. Not listed for UK, AU, NZ and EU and CAN. Listed for USA. http://www.apag.org/issues/methyl.htm#b

E912	$C_{28}H_{56}O_2$ Wax obtained by solvent extraction of lignite (brown coal). Used as a coating for citrus fruits. Listed for UK and EU. Not listed for AU, NZ, CAN and USA.
Montanic acid esters (fat with alcohol). Glazing agent.	
E913 **Lanolin** or **Adeps Lanae** or **Wool wax.** or **Wool grease** Glazing agent, Humectant (water holding).	It is a yellow waxy substance secreted by the sebaceous glands of wool-bearing animals. It is a wax that helps sheep shed water. Certain breeds of sheep produce large amounts of lanolin, and extraction can be performed by squeezing the sheep's harvested wool between rollers. Then it is refined, bleached, deodorized, and dried. Used as an ointment base, for salves and moisturizers for the skin, and in chewing gum. No adverse effects listed in sources. Not listed for UK, AU, NZ and EU. Listed for CAN and USA.
E914	$C_{51}H_{102}O_{21}Si_2$ It is a low molecular weight wax

Oxidized polyethylene wax. Glazing agent.	used in food preparation as a water-impermeable coating for citrus fruits and vegetables. Linked to cancer, kidney and liver damage. Listed for UK, NZ, AU and EU. Not listed for CAN and USA.
E915 **Esters of Colophane.** Glazing agent, Stabilizer.	It is a resin obtained from the pine tree *Pinus silvestris* and related species. Used as a stabilizer in foods and a glazing agent for chewing gum. No adverse effects listed in sources, not much information. Not listed for UK, AU, NZ, USA, EU and CAN.
E916 **Calcium iodate** **or** **Iautarite.** Flour treatment	$Ca(IO_3)_2$. It is a compound of calcium and iodate anion. It is an oxidant added to lotions and ointments as an antiseptic and deodorant. Used in flour, bread and bakery products; used as a dough conditioner. Caution if you have thyroid problems. Not listed for UK, AU, NZ, and EU. Listed for USA and CAN.

agent.	
E917 **Potassium iodate.** Flour treatment agent.	KIO_3 It is a chemical compound that is ionic, made up of K^+ ions and IO_3^- ions in a 1:1 ratio. Sometimes used for iodination of table salt. In some countries, potassium iodate is a source for iodine, lack of iodine is a common deficiency. Can be used to protect against accumulation of radioactive iodine in the thyroid by saturating the body with a stable source of iodine prior to exposure. However, it is not approved by the USA FDA for use as a thyroid blocker. It is highly oxidizing, (causing it to be combine with oxygen). Used in flour, bread and bakery products, also can be an ingredient in baby formula. Caution if you have kidney, heart, or thyroid problems. Not listed for UK, AU, NZ and EU. Listed for CAN and USA.
E918 **Nitrogen oxides.** Preservative, Anti-oxidant.	N_2O (Nitrous oxide) Nitrogen oxide can refer to a binary compound of oxygen and nitrogen, or a mixture of such compounds, as an aerosol spray propellant. Common uses are in aerosol whipped cream canisters, cooking sprays, and inert gas used to displace oxygen. For instance to inhibit bacterial growth, when filling packages of potato chips

	and other similar snack foods. No adverse effects listed in sources. Not listed for UK, NZ, AU and EU. Listed for CAN and USA.
E919 **Nitrogen trichloride** **or** **Trichloramine.** Bleaching agent, Flour treatment agent.	NCl_3 It is made by a combination of ammonium salts, such as ammonium nitrate with chlorine. Used as a bleaching and maturing agent in flour and baked goods. Not much information, no listed bad effects. Not listed for UK, AU, NZ, EU, USA and CAN.
E920 **L-Cysteine monohydro chloride.** Flour treatment	$C_3H_7NO_2S$ It is a non-essential amino acid, which means that it is biosynthesized inside the human body. It is made from animal hair and chicken feathers (80% of world supply). If from China, it may be made from human hair, also can be made synthetically. Used to improve flour and baked goods and to make meat flavors in cube stock. Generally safe if a clean product and used properly.

agent.	Can be a harmful neurotoxin if taken in excess. Listed for UK, NZ, AU, EU and USA. Not listed for CAN.
E921 **L-cysteine hydrochloride monohydrate.** Flour treatment agent.	A different form of L-cysteine, see E920. Not listed for UK, AU, NZ and EU. Listed for CAN.
E922 **Potassium persulfate** **or** **Potassium peroxydisulfate.** Flour	$K_2S_2O_8$ Can be made by electrolysis of a mixture of potassium sulfate and hydrogen sulfate using high current. $2\ KHSO_4 \rightarrow K_2S_2O_8 + H_2$. Used to bleach flour to a white color and to strengthen dough, to allow for higher rising dough. Used in hair dye substances as a whitening agent along with hydrogen peroxide. No adverse effects listed in sources. Not listed for UK, AU, NZ and EU. Listed for CAN and USA.

treatment agent, Bleaching agent.	
E923 **Ammonium persulfate.** Flour treatment agent, Bleaching agent.	$(NH_4)_2S_2O_8$ It is a strong oxidizing agent made synthetically. Used to bleach flour to a white color and to strengthen dough, to allow for a higher rising dough. Used in hair dye substances as a whitening agent along with hydrogen peroxide. No adverse effects listed in sources for ammonium persulfate. Excess ammonia is toxic, but naturally in the body as it is a product of protein catabolism and is safely removed by the liver. Normal blood ammonia levels range from 10-40 µmol/L. People with liver dysfunction may be at increased risk for ammonia toxicity. Early symptoms of ammonia toxicity related to decreasing liver function include inability to concentrate, sleepiness and being prone to irritability. Not listed for UK, AU, NZ and EU. Listed for USA and CAN.
E924	$KBrO_3$ Used to bleach flour to a white color and to strengthen dough to allow higher rising. If used correctly, it is completely used up in the baking

Potassium bromate. Flour treatment agent, Bleaching agent.	process, but if too much or not baked long enough it can leave residues behind that are harmful. Banned in many countries, including EU, Canada, Nigeria, Brazil, Peru, Sri Lanka, and China. Large quantities can cause nausea, vomiting, diarrhoea, abdominal pain, kidney damage and kidney failure, it may be cancer causing. Allowed for use in USA and Japan. The USA FDA has urged bakers to voluntarily stop using it. In California a warning label is required when bromated flour is used. Japanese baked goods manufacturers stopped using potassium bromate voluntarily in 1980; however, Yamazaki Baking resumed its use in 2005, claiming they had new production methods to reduce the amount of the chemical in the final product. (Source Wikipedia). Not listed for UK, NZ, AU, EU and CAN. Listed for USA.
E925 **Chlorine.** Flour treatment agent,	CL It is a chemical element with atomic number 17 and symbol Cl. The element forms diatomic molecules under standard conditions, called dichloride (Cl_2), it is a strong oxidizing agent. The most common compound of chlorine, sodium chloride, has been known since

Bleaching agent.	ancient times, In industry elemental chlorine is usually produced by the electrolysis of sodium chloride dissolved in water. Commonly used in swimming pools, used a flour treatment agent to bleach flour white and to make it stronger for higher rising. Chlorine gas is very harmful to breathe. Chlorine destroys nutrients in foods, a listed carcinogen. Much of the world's public water supply is treated, to make it safer to drink from bacteria (although treatment is not needed in many areas). If home water supply has chlorine in it you can boil water to remove (but goes into the air of the home), or use a filtration system, such as a charcoal filter, also you can install an anti chlorine charcoal filter for the showerhead. There are better alternatives for pool water treatment and spa treatment, for instance using a strong ultraviolet light to kill germs. Not listed for UK, AU, NZ and EU. Listed for CAN and USA.
E926 **Chlorine dioxide**	ClO_2 Over 95% of the chlorine dioxide produced in the world today is made from sodium chlorate. Considered even more effective against germs than ordinary chlorine. Similar as Cl, See E925. Not listed for UK, AU, NZ

or Chlorodioxide **or Chlorine oxide.** Flour treatment agent, Bleaching agent.	and EU. Listed for CAN and USA.
E927a **Azodicarbonamide.** Flour treatment agent, Bleaching agent.	$C_2H_4O_2N_4$ It is a flour treatment and bleaching agent in baked goods, breads, rice, chewing gum, flour and grains. It reacts with moist flour as an oxidizing agent, the USA allows up to 45ppm in flour. It may cause a adverse reaction for those who are also sensitive to azo compounds such as azo food dyes etc. May be a factor for sensitive people to cause or aggravate asthma. Used in products made from flour and baked goods. Not listed for UK, NZ and AU. Listed for USA.
E927b	CH_4N_2O It is commonly known as urea that is found in animal urine. Industrially it is made from ammonia and carbon dioxide. Used as a yeast nutrient in

Carbamide or Urea. Flour treatment agent, Raising agent.	fermented products. It has potential for adverse reactions. Used in teeth whiting products to bleach teeth and also to inhibit potato sprouting, in beer, wine and in baked products. Listed for UK. Not listed for NZ and AU.
E928 Benzoyl peroxide. Flour treatment agent, Bleaching agent.	$C_{14}H_{10}O_4$ It is made by treating benzoyl chloride with barium peroxide. Benzoyl peroxide is used as an acne treatment, for improving flour and for bleaching hair and teeth. It bleaches flour white and increases its strength for rising. Can be used for bleaching out the *carotenoids* (organically based colors) to whiteness. Used in refined flours, cheese, milk, rice and starch. Can be used as an anti acne medicine, but sensitive people may have an adverse reaction on the skin. Asthmatics and people prone to allergies should be cautious. Not listed for UK, AU, NZ and EU. Listed for CAN and USA.
E929 Acetone	$C_6H_{12}O_4$ Or $C_9H_{18}O_6$ It is made by a reaction between hydrogen peroxide and acetone, used in flour products and breads. It is highly explosive in concentrated

peroxide or **Triacetone triperoxide or Peroxyaceto ne or (TATP), (TCAP).** Flour treatment agent, Bleaching agent.	form. It generally burns when ignited and unconfined in quantities less than about 4 grams. More than 4 grams, it will usually detonate when ignited; smaller quantities may detonate when slightly confined. No adverse reactions listed in sources as a food additive, but need more testing. Not listed for UK, NZ, AU and EU and USA. Listed for CAN.
E930 **Calcium peroxide.** Flour treatment agent, Bleaching agent.	CaO_2 It is made by interaction of solutions of calcium salt and sodium peroxide, with subsequent crystallization. Will bleach flour to white, and will make dough stronger so will rise higher. Used in flour, breads, and bakery products. Asthmatics and people with allergies and sensitive have caution. Not listed for UK, AU, NZ and EU. Listed for USA and CAN.

E931 **Nitrogen.** Inert agent for food packing, Preservative.	N2 Elemental nitrogen is a colorless, odorless, tasteless, and mostly inert diatomic gas at standard conditions, constituting 78.08% by volume of earth's atmosphere. Rapid release of nitrogen gas into an enclosed space can displace oxygen, and therefore an asphyxiation hazard. Considered safe as a food packing agent with proper usage. Listed for USA and CAN. Not listed for UK, AU and NZ.
E932 **Nitrous oxide** **or** **Laughing gas** **or** **Sweet air.** Propellant, Inert agent for food packing.	N_2O It is an oxide of nitrogen, the gas is used in surgery and dentistry for its anesthetic and analgesic effects. It is known as laughing gas due to its euphoric effects. It is also used as an oxidizer in rocketry and in motor racing to increase the power output of engines. As a food additive it is used as an aerosol spray propellant for whipped cream canisters, cooking sprays, and as an inert gas used to displace oxygen, to inhibit bacterial growth when filling packages of snack chips and similar packages. It may be used to bleach flour. People (kids) may use the N2O from whipped cream cans to get high. Small amounts are not harmful, but may cause liver, kidney disease and cancer from long term exposure.

	Known to cause damage to fetus in pregnant lab animals. Listed for CAN and USA. Not listed for UK, AU and NZ.
E938 **Argon.** Propellant, Inert agent for food packing.	Ar Argon is the third most common gas in the Earth's atmosphere, at 0.93%. It is an element and inert gas. This element will rarely undergo any kind of chemical reactions. It has a complete octet (eight electrons) in the outer atomic shell making argon stable and resistant to bonding with other elements. Can be used in packing foods and in arasol cans as a propellant. A main use is as a shielding gas for welding. In large quantities it can displace oxygen, because it is 25% more heavy (dense) than air so will stay down low in enclosed spaces making it dangerous. Safe with proper usage. Listed for UK and EU. Not listed for NZ, AU and CAN and USA.
E939 **Helium.** Propellant,	He It is the chemical element with atomic number 2 and an atomic weight of 4.002602; it has two protons and two neutrons. An inert gas so it is rarely reactive. It is lighter than air so not extremely dangerous in displacing air, but still need caution in enclosed spaces. Will

Inert agent for food packing.	cause a high pitch voice when breathed, and too much can cause asphyxiation. Can be used as a propellant in canisters and as an inert gas in snack packages. Considered safe with proper usage. Listed for UK, USA and EU. Not listed for AU, NZ and CAN.
E940 **Dichlorodifluoromethane, or (common brand name) Freon-12.** Propellant, Anti-freeze.	CCl_2F_2 It is a synthetic inert gas. Used as a propellant, and anti-freeze in canned and frozen products. It is used in air-conditioning units. Damaging to the ozone layer, so it is banned in most countries and hardly used these days. Not listed for UK, AU, NZ and CAN. Listed for USA.
E941 **Nitrogen.** Inert agent for food packing, Freezing agent.	N It is a chemical element that has the symbol N, atomic number of 7 and atomic mass 14.00674. It is mostly inert, normally N2 in nature a very hard bond to break and very stable. There is an asphyxiation hazard if N2 gas is in an enclosed space. In liquid form it can cause freezer burns on skin. Nitrogen also dissolves in the bloodstream and body fats. Rapid decompression (in particular, in the

	case of divers ascending too quickly, or astronauts decompressing too quickly from cabin pressure to spacesuit pressure) can lead to a potentially fatal condition called decompression sickness (Bends). As a food additive, it is used as an antioxidant in food packages, also used in freezing and vacuum packing, seems safe in proper usage. Listed for UK, AU, NZ, USA, EU and CAN.
E942 **Nitrous oxide.** Propellant.	Inert agent for food packing, similar as E932, see E932. Listed for UK, NZ, AU, EU, USA and CAN.
E943a **Butane.** Propellant.	C_4H_{10} Isomer of Iso-butane meaning same molecular structure, but different shape. Propellant used in spray cans and foam products, also used in refrigeration systems. Mildly toxic if inhaled, a neurotoxin in high dosages. May be cancer causing. Generally safe with proper usage. Listed for AU, UK, NZ, USA, EU and CAN.

E943b **Iso-butane.** Propellant.	C_4H_{10} Isomer of butane, meaning same molecular structure, but different shape. Propellant used in spray cans and foam products also used in refrigeration systems. Mildly toxic if inhaled, a neurotoxin in high dosages. May be cancer causing. Generally safe with proper usage. Listed for UK, AU, NZ, EU, USA and CAN.
E944 **Propane.** Propellant.	C_3H_8 A by-product of natural gas processing and petroleum refining, it is commonly used as a fuel for engines, oxy-gas torches, barbecues, portable stoves, and home heating. Propane is denser than air, so it tends to sink and stay inside any enclosed area, it may cause explosion and fire. For safety propane tanks should be used and stored outside if possible away from housing structures. Propellant used in spray cans. It may be a narcotic and neurotoxin in high amounts. Listed for UK, AU, NZ, USA, EU and CAN.
E945 **Chloropenta fluoroethan**	C_2ClF_5 It is a chlorofluorocarbon once used as a refrigerant, this use has been banned since 1 January 1996 because of its ozone-depleting action. Also once used as a propellant in

e. Propellant.	aerosol cans. Not listed in UK, EU, AU and NZ. Listed for CAN and USA.
E946 **Octafluoroc yclobutane.** Propellant.	C_4F_8, May be used as a refrigerant in specialized applications, as a replacement for ozone depleting chlorofluorocarbon refrigerants. It may be used as a propellant in aerosol foods and whipped creams etc. It is investigated as a possible replacement for sulfur hexafluoride as a dielectric gas. More study needed for health, caution. Not listed for UK and EU. Listed for AU, NZ, USA and CAN.
E948 **Oxygen.** Packaging gas.	O Oxygen is an element with atomic number 8 (8 protons) and represented by the symbol O. It is normally in a diatomic state O2 when in pure form as a gas. As a food additive it is a packaging gas for fresh vegetables, and meat, it makes the meat bright red in color which is appealing without using coloring. No harmful effects when used for food packaging. Fire hazard and explosive, do not let high pressure O2 gas spray on petroleum products (for instance on grease in pipe fittings) if so will

	cause fire or explosion. Listed for UK and EU. Not listed for AU, NZ, CAN and USA.
E949 **Hydrogen.** Packaging gas.	H It is the chemical element with atomic number 1 (one proton). It is normally in a diatomic state H2 when in pure form as a gas. Used as a packaging gas to prevent spoilage and oxidation of foods. No harmful effects noted in sources when used in food packaging. Fire hazard and explosive. Listed for UK and EU. Not listed for AU, NZ, CAN and USA.
E950 **Acesulfame potassium** **or** **Acesulfame K** **or** **Ace K** **(marketed under the trade names Sunett and Sweet One).**	$C_4H_4KNO_4S$ It is industrially made by the synthetic transformation of acetoacetic acid in combination with potassium to form a white crystalline powder. It can be used in most any product as a sweetener. Acesulfame K is 180-200 times sweeter than table sugar, as sweet as aspartame, half as sweet as saccharin, and one-quarter as sweet as sucralose. It has a slightly bitter aftertaste especially in high concentration. Acesulfame K is often blended with other sweeteners, usually sucralose or aspartame. This gives a better tasting product with a sugar like taste and little to no aftertaste. Possible cancer causing agent as it causes cancer in animals,

Artificial sweetener.	it also causes high cholesterol in animals. It may cause low blood sugar attacks for sensitive people. Listed for UK, AU, NZ, EU, USA and CAN.
E951 **Aspartame.** **(Sold under brand name NutraSweet and later sold under the brand name AminoSweet).** Artificial sweetener.	$C_{14}H_{18}N_2O_5$ Aspartame is a methyl ester of the dipeptide of the natural amino acids L-aspartic acid and L-phenylalanine, it is chemically made and not natural. It is about 200 times sweeter than table sugar with a longer lasting sweet aftertaste. It can be used in most any food and there is a long list of these in use including soda. It can be combined with other sweeteners for better taste and product stability. It is often used for diet products, but can be found in any processed product. It is in thousands of different products. It naturally breaks down to formaldehyde in the body, shown in recent independent studies to accumulate in the protein of organs and muscles of test animals, even in low dosages. As of 1995 when the U.S. Food and Drug Administration (FDA) was quoted as saying they stopped accepting adverse reaction reports on aspartame, it is noted that over 75% of the adverse reactions were due to aspartame. It is likely that there are

millions of examples of aspartame toxicity reactions. Toxicity symptoms reported include seizures, headaches, memory loss, tremors, convulsions, vision loss, nausea, dizziness, confusion, depression, irritability, anxiety attacks, personality changes, heart palpitations, chest pains, skin diseases, loss of blood sugar control, arthritic symptoms, weight gain (in some cases, as per an addictive condition), fluid retention, excessive thirst or urination. On going ingestion may cause chronic diseases such as cancer. It is a slowly accumulating sort of toxin, but it can cause acute reactions as well. Avoid if pregnant.

As a practical matter, the largest danger is an ongoing ingestion of any product that causes an adverse reaction. I know of someone who drank a soda product with aspartame for a long period of time and it seemed to have a harmful effect (couldn't hardly walk then stopped drinking it and in about two weeks they were able to walk much better). It is odd, but often an item people have an adverse reaction to, they also have an addictive feeling for it as well. *Studies show high levels of*

	aspartame may trigger a craving for carbohydrates by depleting the brain of a chemical that registers carbohydrate satiety. This can lead to weight gain while using low calorie diet food and drink products. http://www.mbm.net.au/health/worst_additives.htm Listed for UK, AU, NZ, EU, USA and CAN.
E952 **Salts of Cyclamic acid or** **Sodium cyclamate or Calcium cyclamate.** Artificial sweetener.	$C_6H_{12}NNaO_3S$ They are chemically made from cyclohexylsulfamic acid to form an odorless white crystalline powder. Sodium cyclamate is 30–50 times sweeter than sugar. Used in drinks, dry drinks mixes, sugars, sugar preserves, jams, jellies, low-calorie frozen desserts, soft drinks, chewing gum, and baked goods etc. Often used with saccharin to improve sweetness and shelf life. The mixture of 10 parts cyclamate to 1 part saccharin is common and masks the off-tastes of both sweeteners. Shown to cause cancer, also embryo and testicular problems in mice/rats may cause similar problems in humans. Known to cause headaches, migraines, and other reactions in people. May be in foods illegally in excessive amounts. Listed for UK, AU, NZ, EU. Not listed for CAN and

	USA(banned).
E953 **Isomalt or Isomaltitol.** Artificial sweetener.	$C_{12}H_{24}O_{11}$ Isomalt is a disaccharide composed of the two sugars glucose and mannitol. Most likely to be made from beets, source carbohydrate for Isomalt may be from genetically modified plants. Can be used in many foods and drinks. Considered suitable for diabetics, as it does not have a large effect on blood glucose or serum insulin levels. Can cause softer than normal stool and intestinal gas if used in excess Not permitted in infant foods. Considered safe in proper usage for most people in listed sources. Listed for UK, AU, NZ, EU and CAN. Not listed for USA.
E954 **Saccharin.** Artificial sweetener.	$C_7H_5NO_3S$ It is chemically made by the oxidation of o-toluenesulfonamide. It can be used in many foods and drinks. It is 200-700 times sweeter than sugar with a bitter metallic after taste, especially when used in high concentration. A 10:1 cyclamate :saccharin blend is common where legal to mask the off taste of each. Saccharin is often used together with aspartame in diet sodas, because aspartame has a shorter shelf life. Even though it has no food energy, it

	can cause the release of insulin. In its acid form saccharin is not water-soluble. The form used as an artificial sweetener is usually its sodium salt form. There is controversy over this artificial sweetener. Original studies show it causes cancer in rodents (bladder and reproductive cancers), but recent thought is that the mechanism for cancer for rodents does not exist for humans. Other sources indicate it still may cause cancer in humans. Caution, use in extreme moderation. It was listed then de listed then listed back in various countries(USA) for use and the controversy continues. Banned in many countries. Listed for UK, AU, NZ, EU and USA. Not listed for CAN.
E955 **Sucralose** **(Can be found under brand name "Splenda").** Artificial sweetener.	$C_{12}H_{19}Cl_3O_8$ It is manufactured by the selective chlorination of sucrose (table sugar), which substitutes three of the hydroxyl groups with chloride, it may be chemically made without sugar. It is about 600 times sweeter than table sugar, twice as sweet as saccharin, and 3.3 times as sweet as aspartame. It is used in thousands of foods and drinks to make them sweeter. It can be used in combination with other sweeteners. In animal studies, it caused a shrunken thymus gland,

	enlarged liver and kidneys, miscarriages. It can have traces of heavy metals and other toxins. Those with chlorine allergies may have adverse reaction. Linked to bladder and reproductive cancers in animal studies. Listed for UK, AU, NZ, EU, USA and CAN.
E956 **Alitame (Can be found under brand name "Aclame.").** Artificial sweetener.	$C_{14}H_{25}N_3O_4S$ Like aspartame, alitame is an aspartic acid-containing dipeptide. It is about 2000 times sweeter than table sugar and about 10 times sweeter than aspartame. Very stable over wide ranges of temperature and Ph which gives products longer shelf life. May be used in thousands of different foods and beverage products. It increased liver weight during testing with animals when given high amounts, needs more research. Not listed for UK, USA, CAN and EU. Listed for AU and NZ.
E957 **Thaumatin.** Artificial sweetener, Flavor	Thaumatin is a low-calorie sweetener and flavor modifier. It is a natural protein, is used primarily for its flavor-modifying properties rather than a single lone sweetener. Used to sweeten wines, chewing gum, bread and fruit etc. Some of the proteins in the thaumatin family are natural sweeteners roughly 2000 times more potent than sugar. Although very

enhancer.	sweet, thaumatin's taste is very different from sugar. The sweetness of thaumatin builds very slowly and perception lasts a long time, leaving a liquorice-like aftertaste with a concentrated amount. Used with other artificial sweeteners to improve taste in some way, for instance it masks Saccharin's after taste. Not to be used in infant foods, needs more research, caution. Listed for UK, AU, NZ, USA, CAN, EU, Israel and Japan.
E958 Glycyrrhizin Artificial sweetener, Flavor enhancer, Foaming agent.	$C_{42}H_{62}O_{16}$ It is the main sweet-tasting compound from liquorice root. It is 30–50 times sweeter than table sugar. The sweetness of glycyrrhizin has a slower onset than sugar, and lingers in the mouth. It can be used as medicine for treatment of ulcers in the gastrointestinal track and as an expectorant (clears mucus from lungs or nasal cavities etc). Possible side effects are water retention and high blood pressure-due to the effect on kidneys. Listed for EU, USA and Japan. Not listed for UK, NZ, AU, CAN and EU.
E959	$C_{28}H_{36}O_{15}$ It is commercially made by extracting neohesperidin from citrus fruit mostly oranges and then

Neohesperidine dihydrochalcone or Neohesperidin DC or **NHDC.** Artificial sweetener, Flavor enhancer.	hydrogenating neohesperidin. It is about 340 times sweeter than sugar when compared by weight; it has a relatively long shelf life, up to five years in good conditions. In food it is used as a flavor enhancer in concentrations of around 4-5 parts per million (ppm) and as an artificial sweetener at around 15-20 ppm. This is well below one percent so may not be on food label. It is combined with other sweeteners with good effect such as aspartame, saccharin, acesulfame potassium, cyclamate, and xylitol. It is in many foods and beverages, anything that needs a sweetener. At a concentration of 20 ppm, NHDC can produce side effects such as nausea and migraine. Listed for UK and EU. Not listed for AU, NZ, CAN and USA.
E960 **Stevioside.** Artificial sweetener, Flavor enhancer.	$C_{20}H_{30}O_3$ Extracted from the leaves of the stevia plant, it is about 300 times sweeter than table sugar. Safe for diabetics because it will not cause a glycemic response. It can be used in many foods and beverages. Stevia has been safely used for hundreds of years and there are no commonly known bad side effects, but nevertheless monitor yourself while using and use in moderation. Listed

	for UK, AU and NZ, EU. Not listed for CAN and USA.
E961 **Neotame.** Artificial sweetener, Flavor enhancer.	$C_{20}H_{30}N_2O_5$ Made of the amino acids aspartic acid and phenylalanine, to form a white to off-white powder, it is between 7,000 and 13,000 times sweeter than table sugar. It can be used in any kind of food and beverage as a flavor enhancer. It is very economical to use because very little is needed. In pure form it can have a bitter aftertaste like most artificial sweeteners. Many industry-sponsored studies show that it is safe, but there is much controversy because it is chemically similar to aspartame. Caution until more time has passed and more independent studies are completed. Listed for AU, NZ, UK, USA, EU, AU and NZ. Not listed for CAN.
E962 **Aspartame-acesulfame salt,** **(Marketed under the name**	$C_{18}H_{23}O_9N_3S$ It is made by soaking a 2 to 1 mixture of aspartame and acesulfame potassium in an acidic solution and allowing it to crystallize. It is about 350 times sweeter than table sugar. It is a salt of Aspartame, caution, see E951. Allowed in EU, USA, AU and New Zealand. Listed for UK, AU, NZ and EU. Not listed for CAN and USA.

Twinsweet). Artificial sweetener, Flavor enhancer.	
E965 **Maltitol or** **Maltitol syrup or Hydrogenat ed glucose syrup, (It is also known under trade names, Maltisorb, Maltisweet and Lesys).** Sugar alcohol sweetener, Flavor enhancer.	$C_{12}H_{24}O_{11}$ Maltitol is made by hydrogenation of maltose obtained from starch (source starch may come from genetically modified plants). It has about 90 percent the sweetness of table sugar. Used in production of sugar free sweets such as sugarless hard candies, chewing gum, chocolates, baked goods, and ice cream. May cause gastrointestinal distress or digestion upset especially if eaten in excess; it is a laxative in high amounts (more than 100 grams in a day). Sugar alcohols can covert to fat and may contribute to high triglycerides, therefore cause heart disease and weight gain, may cause carbohydrate cravings- all depending on personal eating habits and genetics. Listed for UK, AU, USA, EU and NZ.

E966 Lactitol. Sugar alcohol sweetener, Flavor enhancer.	$C_{12}H_{24}O_{11}$ It is made by the hydrogenation of lactose derived from whey (milk) it is a sugar alcohol. It has about 40% the sweetness of table sugar; it is often combined with more powerful artificial sweeteners. High stability makes it popular for baking. Used in sugar-free candies, cookies, chocolates, and ice cream. It can be used as a laxative. For some people it may cause intestinal cramping, flatulence, and diarrhea. The dosage recommended to fight constipation is 10 grams, it is easy to eat more than this with some kinds of sweets, beware a possible laxative effect with over 20g per day. Sugar alcohols can covert to fat and may contribute to high triglycerides, therefore cause heart disease and weight gain (may cause carbohydrate cravings), all depending on personal eating habits and genetics. Listed for UK, NZ, AU, EU and CAN. Not listed for USA.
E967 **Xylitol.**	$C_5H_{12}O_5$ Industrially it is made from birch trees with other hard wood trees and fibrous vegetables. About as sweet as table sugar with only two-thirds the food energy. Used in chewing gum and other sweets, can be used in most any food product, also used in

Sugar alcohol sweetener, Flavor enhancer, Humectant (holds water), Stabilizer, Bulking agent.	toothpastes and mouthwashes. For some people it may cause intestinal cramping, flatulence, and diarrhea especially if eaten in excess. Notable effect for children if more than 65 grams a day (4 out of 13 with negative effects). Sugar alcohols can covert to fat, and may contribute to high triglycerides, therefore cause heart disease risk and weight gain (may cause carbohydrate cravings), all depending on personal eating habits and genetics. Listed for UK, AU, NZ, EU, USA and CAN. http://www.annualreviews.org/doi/abs/10.1146/annurev.nu.01.070181.002253
E968 **Erythritol.** Sugar alcohol sweetener, Flavor enhancer, Humectant (holds water).	$C_4H_{10}O_4$ Industrially it is made from glucose by fermentation with yeast, *Moniliella pollinis*. It is 60–70% as sweet as table sugar and is almost non-caloric. It has a clean cool taste with no aftertaste. It is often used with other ingredients to improve food texture, moisture content, to inhibit crystallization, and to counteract its cooling effects. It can be used with other sweeteners. Used in candy, chocolate, yogurt, jellies, beverages, and as a sugar substitute. It is considered to be better tolerated than other sugar alcohols because

	90% of erythritol is absorbed before it enters the large intestine, so it does not normally cause laxative effects like other sugar alcohols. Sugar alcohols can covert to fat, and may contribute to high triglycerides. Therefore may cause heart disease and weight gain (carbohydrate cravings), all depending on personal eating habits and genetics. Listed for UK, AU, NZ, EU and CAN. Not listed for USA.
E999 **Quillaia extract.** Foaming agent, Hemectant (water holding agent).	$C_{30}H_{46}O_5$ Quillaia is the milled inner bark or small stems and branches of the quillaia tree (called the "soap bark tree" because of the soapy foam the bark can produce). It is native to Peru and Chile, and cultivated in Northern Hindustan. The extract is used as a foaming agent in beverages mostly in soft drinks and in some sports drinks. It is also used as a humectant (water holding agent) in baked goods and frozen dairy products etc. The initial extract is non-toxic, but can break down into toxic elements. The extract can be used medicinally as an expectorant (pushes mucus out of the chest). Caution, it is banned in many countries. Listed for UK, EU and USA. Not listed for AU, NZ and CAN.

E1000 **Cholic acid** Emulsifier (mixing and blending agent).	$C_{24}H_{40}O_5$ Cholic acid is a bile acid (acids found in the bile of mammals). Salts of cholic acid are called cholates. It is extracted from the bile of cows, but for industry it likely produced synthetically. Emulsifier used to make dry egg powder. Acceptable daily intake is up to 1.25 mg per kg of bodyweight. No negative effect reported in sources, but seldom used in foods. Not listed in UK, AU, NZ, EU and CAN. Listed for USA.
E1001 **Choline salts.** Emulsifier (mixing and blending agent), B Vitamin.	$C_5\,H_{14}\,N\,O$ Choline is a water-soluble essential nutrient meaning the human body cannot make it. Choline is usually grouped within the B-complex of vitamins. Vegetarians, vegans, endurance athletes, and people who drink a lot of alcohol or diuretics (excessive tea or coffee etc) are at an extra risk for choline deficiency. Overall vitamin B deficiency is common. Used as emulsifier in many foods such as fat spreads, processed fruits, breakfast cereals, pre-cooked pastas, baked goods, chocolates and soybean based products etc. Choline supplementation is good in general, but be cautious of synthetic vitamins, also of imbalances of vitamins-either

	too much or too little of any single vitamin in relation to others. Not listed in UK, EU and CAN. Listed for AU, NZ and USA.
E1100 **Amylase.** Flour treatment agent, (Enzyme), Raising agent.	$C_{36}H_{55}NO_{28}$ It is made from mold mushroom or pig pancreas, it is an enzyme that helps break down starches into sugars. Amylase is naturally present in human saliva, where it begins the chemical process of digestion. Used as an additive for bread making to cause starches in flour to break down, so the bread will rise because of CO_2 production. Used in baked products, no known bad effects noted in sources. Not listed for UK and EU. Listed for AU, NZ, USA and CAN.
E1101 **Proteases.** Flour treatment agent. (enzyme), Raising agent.	Naturally, in the human body, it breaks down proteins for digestion. As an additive it breaks down proteins into amino acids. It is used to prepare flour and dough for baking, also in beer and other alcoholic beverages. It is an exotoxin creator (a toxin excreted by a microorganism), that may cause cellular damage. Some proteases may have teratogenic properties (causes abnormal development of children). May be genetically modified, caution. Not listed in UK and EU. Listed for AU, NZ, USA and CAN.

E1102 **Glucose oxidase.** Anti-oxidant, Anti-microbial agent, Preservative.	It is a enzyme made from genetically modified fungi that prevents spoilage due to oxidation. It is naturally found in honey. No known common usages to date and not much information in sources. Not listed in UK and EU. Listed for CAN, AU, NZ and USA.
E1103 **Invertase.** Enzyme (Increases rate of reaction), Flavoring agent.	$C_{12}H_{24}O_{12}$ Commercially invertase is made from yeast; it is an enzyme that aids the break down of sucrose (table sugar). The result is a mixture of fructose and glucose that is called "inverted sugar syrup" (a mixture of glucose and fructose, which is made by splitting sucrose into these two components). Inverted sugar syrup is sweeter than sugar and its products tend to remain more moist and less prone to crystallization. It is mainly used in sweets and candies, not much information, but seems safe. Invertase is relativity expensive so not in much use, there are cheaper ways to make inverted sugar syrup.

	Listed for UK, EU, USA and CAN. Not listed for AU and NZ.
E1104 **Lipases.** Enzyme (Increases rate of reaction), Flavoring agent, Emulsifier (mixing agent), Flour treatment agent.	Lipase is made from many kinds of fungi, which may be genetically modified. There are many kinds of lipases and they help break down lipids (fats). Lipases are natural in the human body and in the animal kingdom. Used in fermented products such as yogurt, cheeses, soy sauces and derivatives of these, in baked goods, egg products and oil. Not much information in listed sources, but appears relatively safe. Not listed in UK, EU and USA. Listed for AU, NZ and CAN.
E1105 **Lysozyme** Enzyme (Increases rate of	$C_{15}H_{20}O_4$ It is a enzyme that is naturally inside tears, saliva, blood and (human) milk. It is an important part of the immune system defense for humans and animals. It is industrially prepared from chicken eggs or by bacteria. If babies are fed lysozyme deficient baby formula, their immune systems will be weaker. It is mostly used in European semi hard cheeses to prevent spoliation of cheese when

reaction), Preservative, Anti bacterial agent.	maturing. Used for infant nutrition and other pharmaceutical preparations; no noted bad effects in sources with proper usage. Listed for AU, NZ, USA and CAN. Not listed for UK and EU.
E1200 **Polydextrose.** Humectant (Water holding agent), Stabilizing agent, Thickening agent.	(C6H10O5)n Polydextrose is an indigestible synthetic polymer of glucose Made by heating dextrose (glucose) in the presence of sorbitol and citric acid. It is often used to increase the fiber content of food-may not be as healthy as natural fiber found in foods. It is a modifying agent used in baked foods, confectionary, chocolate, jam, ice cream and low calorie foods. Binds with water and protects against freeze damage, it is considered suitable for diabetics. Fat substitute that may be corn based (Source corn may be genetically modified). Polydextrose in excess may cause gastrointestinal upset and have a laxative effect. Listed for UK, AU, NZ, EU, USA and CAN.
E1201 **Polyvinylpyrrolidone or Polyvidone or**	(C6H9NO)n May cause cancer, lung and kidney damage; liver toxicity, allergic reactions, skin reactions. gas and fecal impaction or constipation. Supposed to be inert and non toxic. Made from acetylene, hydrogen,

Povidone. Stabilizing agent, Thickening agent, Glazing agent (to coat pills, etc).	formaldehyde and ammonia. Used in flavors and fragrances, pharmaceuticals, as coating for tablets. Used in artificial sweeteners, low calorie foods and gum. May want to avoid especially in excess. Listed for UK, USA, EU and CAN. Not listed for AU and NZ.
E1202 **Polyvinylpolypyrrolidon eor Polyvinyl polypyrrolidone or PVPP or Crospovidone or Crospolividone.** Stabilizing agent, Color retention agent, Clarifying agent, Sweetener.	$C6H9NO)n$ It is a highly cross-linked modification of polyvinylpyrrolidone (PVP) see E1201. Insoluble in water, but will absorb water. As a clarifying agent it will absorb compounds out of solution, useful for wine and beer making. It also can be used as a sweetener in many kinds of foods and beverages. Used in beer and malt beverages, white wine, cider and water-based flavored drinks, dairy-base drinks, chewing gum, tabletop sweetener, glazing for fruit, cream, condensed milk, cheese, dairy based dessert and cereals, etc. Mostly unabsorbed when taken orally, but it can damage kidneys and take up to a year before the body can totally remove it, best to avoid. Listed for UK, USA, EU and CAN. Not listed for AU and NZ.
E1204	$(C_6H_{12}O_5)_n$ Pullulan is a natural polysaccharide made from starch by fermentation of

Pullulan. Thickening agent, Coating agent.	a fungus. The source starch may be from genetically modified plants. Used as a coating agent on baked goods and on candies as a decoration. Also used in breath fresheners, mouth wash products and as pill coatings. Pullulanase, which is a enzyme created by genetically modified bacteria will hydrolytically cleave pullulan. Some adverse effects noted in rodent studies. Not much information. http://whqlibdoc.who.int/publications/2006/9241660562_part1_d_eng.pdf Listed for UK and EU. Not listed for AU, NZ, CAN and USA.
E1205 **Basic methacrylate copolymer.** Coating agent.	Can be used as a coating agent on supplements and pills etc. Synthetically made. http://www.ncbi.nlm.nih.gov/pubmed/21704668 http://www.efsa.europa.eu/de/efsajournal/pub/1513.htm Some studies indicate that is safe, but not much information. Listed for UK.

E1400 to E1450

Modified starches, are made by various processes, physically or enzymatically or chemically in order to change their natural properties. Modified starches are used in all starch applications, as thickening agents, stabilizing agents or emulsifying agents, in commercial food products and pharmaceuticals.

Starches are modified to improve their natural condition in different applications. Starches may be modified to increase their stability against excessive heat, acid, shear, time, cooling, or freezing; in order to change texture, to decrease or increase their viscosity and to lengthen or shorten gelatinization time.

Can be made from genetically modified sources (corn). Additional possible danger is traces of the modifying chemical (if used) being left behind

| **E1400** **Dextrin** Stabilizing agent, Thickening agent, Binding agent | $(C_6H_{10}O_5)_n$ It is made commercially by applying dry heat under acidic conditions, a way of roasting. It is a partially hydrolyzed starch; the source starch may be wheat or corn-if corn may be genetically modified. It is a polymer of dextrose, a manmade substance made from starch. Can be used in many products including flavored milks, whipped creams, whey products, fat-based desserts, coffee substitutes, confectionary, hot cereal, breakfast oats, pre-cooked pastas and noodles, batters, starch based desserts (rice pudding, tapioca), pie fillings, sauces, salad dressings, soups, puddings and custards, it can be in infant foods. May cause adverse |

	reactions for sensitive people, people with celiac disease should avoid. It needs more research, caution. Not listed in UK, EU and CAN. Listed for AU, NZ and USA.
E1401 **Acid treated starch.** Stabilizing agent, Thickening agent, Binding agent.	Made by immersing starch with acid such as sulfuric acid, hydrochloric acid, or phosphoric acid, afterward it is neutralized by sodium hydroxide or sodium carbonate. Used in many processed foods to bind or thicken or to stabilize foods. Can be used in many products including flavored milks, whipped creams, whey products, fat-based desserts, coffee substitutes , confectionary, hot cereal, breakfast oats, pre-cooked pastas and noodles, batters, starch based desserts (rice pudding, tapioca), pie fillings, sauces, salad dressings, soups, puddings, and custards etc. No known adverse effects noted in sources. Not listed for UK, EU and CAN. Listed for AU, NZ and USA.
E1402 **Alkaline modified starch.**	It is made by treating starch with sodium or potassium hydroxide. The starch is somewhat degraded; can be used in many products including flavored milks, whipped creams, whey products, fat-based desserts, coffee substitutes, confectionary, hot cereal, breakfast oats, pre-cooked

Stabilizing agent, Thickening agent, Binding agent.	pastas and noodles, batters, starch based desserts (rice pudding, tapioca), pie fillings, sauces, salad dressings, soups, puddings and custards etc No adverse effects noted in sources, not much information. Not listed for UK, EU, USA and CAN. Listed for AU and NZ.
E1403 **Bleached starch** Stabilizing agent, Thickening agent, Binding agent.	Bleached starch is made by treating starch with bleaching chemicals such as hydrogen peroxide, which oxidizes the starch. Source starch may be genetically modified (i.e. GE corn). This process removes any distasteful colors in the starch and leaves it mostly unchanged for usage in processed foods. Can be used in many products including flavored milks, whipped creams, whey products, fat-based desserts, coffee substitutes, confectionary, hot cereal, breakfast oats, pre-cooked pastas and noodles, batters, starch based desserts (rice pudding, tapioca), pie fillings, sauces, salad dressings, soups, puddings and custards etc. May cause asthmatics an asthma attack because it may be treated with sulfur dioxide. Not listed for UK, CAN and EU. Listed for AU, NZ and USA.
E1404	It is made from starch and sodium hypochlorite, breaking down the

Oxidized starch. Stabilizing agent, Thickening agent, Binding agent.	starch and decreasing its natural viscosity. One use is in batters to help them better stick to fish and meat, and in candies to increase shelf life and clarity, and to improve taste in many products. May have sulfur dioxide residue, which is dangerous to asthmatics. High concentrations cause diarrhea and kidney defects in animals. It needs more study, caution. Listed for UK, AU, NZ, EU and USA. Not listed for CAN.
E1405 **Enzyme treated starch, Maltodextrin, and Cyclodextrin.** Stabilizing agent, Thickening agent, Binding agent.	Made by treating starch with enzymes; the two kinds of starch are maltodextrin, and cyclodextrin. These are partially broken down to have a lower viscosity. Can be used in many products including flavored milks, whipped creams, whey products, fat-based desserts, coffee substitutes , confectionary, hot cereal, breakfast oats, pre-cooked pastas and noodles, batters, starch based desserts (rice pudding, tapioca), pie fillings, sauces, salad dressings, soups, puddings and custards. Thickener, vegetable gum used in baby foods etc. Starch may come from genetically modified plants (corn). Adverse reactions are possible for sensitive people and celiacs should avoid. Not listed for UK, EU and CAN. Listed for AU, NZ

	and USA.
E1410 **Mono-starch phosphate.** Stabilizing agent, Thickening agent, Binding agent.	Mono starch phosphate is made with phosphorous acid or the salts sodium phosphate, potassium phosphate, or sodium triphosphate. This causes the starch to break down, to be less viscose. The resulting starch is partially degraded and phosphorylated. Most common uses are batters for frozen foods, puddings, desserts, sauces, pies and fillings, mayonnaise, salad dressings, instant beverages and dried foods. Also used in many other products. Source starch may be from genetically modified plant sources. (GM corn) No adverse reactions reported in listed sources. Listed for UK, AU, NZ and EU. Not listed for CAN and USA.
E1411 **Distarch glycerol.** Stabilizing agent, Thickening agent,	Distarch glycerol is made by treating starch with glycerol. The starch is partially degraded and combined with glycerol. Most common uses are batters for frozen foods, puddings, desserts, sauces, pies and fillings, mayonnaise, salad dressings, instant beverages and dried foods. Also used in many other products. No adverse effects listed in sources. Not listed for UK, AU, NZ, CAN and EU. Listed for USA.

Emulsifier (mixing agent).	
E1421 **Starch Acetate Esterified with Vinyl Acetate.** Stabilizing agent, Thickening agent, Emulsifier (mixing agent), Binding agent.	It is made by treating starch with vinyl acetate. The resulting starch is more stable at a higher temperature and lower pH (acidic). Similar to E1420. Used in many kinds of foods, but mostly for frozen foods such as ice creams, soy ice creams and frozen cakes. Also used in confectionary, yoghrts, egg white mix and fruit flavored fillings etc. May be made from genetically modified plants. May cause diarrhea, and needs more testing. Not listed for AU, UK, NZ, CAN and EU. Listed for USA.
E1422 **Acelylated distarch adipate.** Stabilizing agent,	It is made by treating starch with acetic acid anhydride and adipinic acid anhydride. This makes a modified starch that is resistant against stirring and high temperatures. This starch is used as a thickener in a wide range of foods such as relishes and pickles, fruit pies and fillings and baby food. May be made from genetically modified plants. It has no known adverse

Thickening agent, Emulsifier (mixing agent), Binding agent.	effects with low amounts, but further testing is needed. (Animal tests showed slowed growth rates and renal lesions.). Listed for UK, AU, NZ, USA and EU. Not listed for CAN.
E1423 **Acetylated distarch glycerol.** Stabilizing agent, Thickening agent, Emulsifier (mixing agent), Binding agent.	It is made by treating starch with acetic acid anhydride and glycerol. This makes a starch more resistant against stirring and increased stability for high temperatures and after cooling. Used in frozen cakes, dry mixes and sauces, breakfast cereals, pies, custard powders, mayonnaises, salad dressings, infant foods and many others. May be made from genetically modified plants. No adverse effects listed in sources. Not listed for UK, AU, NZ, CAN and EU. Listed for USA.
E1430 **Distarch**	Distarch glycerine is made by treating starch with glycerol. This causes the starch to partly breakdown (hydrolyze). Then it is more stable against heat, acids,

glycerine. Stabilizing agent, Thickening agent, Emulsifier (mixing agent).	alkalis and starch degrading enzymes. Used in batters for frozen foods, desserts, custards, sauces, mayonnaise, salad dressings, puddings, pies, fillings and dried foods. May be made from genetically modified plants. Not much information, no adverse effects noted in sources. Not listed for UK, AU, NZ, CAN, USA and EU.
E1440 **Hydroxypropyl starch** Stabilizing agent, Thickening agent, Emulsifier (mixing agent).	It is made by treating starch with propyleneoxide, then it is more stable against heat, acids, alkalis and starch degrading enzymes. Mostly used in frozen foods, ice-cream, soy ice-cream, frozen cakes, dry mixes, flavored toppings, sauces and gravies and more. May be made from genetically modified plants, no adverse effects noted in sources. Listed for UK, AU, NZ, EU and USA. Not listed for CAN.
E1441	Made by treating starch with propyleneoxide, epichlorhydrine and glycerol. Then it is more stable

Hydroxy propyl distarch glycerine. Stabilizing agent, Thickening agent, Emulsifier (mixing agent).	against acid, alkaline and starch degrading enzymes. This modified starch also provides better color, shine to products and is more stable after cooling. May be made from genetically modified plants. May cause diarrhea, not much information. Not listed for UK, AU, NZ, CAN, USA and EU.
E1442 **Hydroxy propyl distarch phosphate.** Stabilizing agent, Thickening agent, Emulsifier (mixing	It is made by treating starch with propyleneoxide and phosphoric acid. Then the starch is more stable against acid, alkaline and starch degrading enzymes. It is also more stable for freeze/thaw cycles. Mostly used in frozen foods, ice-cream, soy ice-cream, frozen cakes, dry mixes, flavored toppings, sauces, gravies and many more. May be made from genetically modified plants, may slow down digestion, it needs more testing. No adverse effects noted in sources. Listed for UK, AU, NZ, EU and USA. Not listed for CAN.

agent).	
E1450 **Starch sodium octenyl succinate.** Thickening agent, Emulsifier (mixing agent).	It is made by treating starch with octenylsuccinate, makes it good for products containing oil-in-water emulsions (an emulsifier). It is easily soluble in cold liquids. It effectively disperses oils and fats in sauces and stays stable, unchanging when food is frozen and thawed and extends the shelf life of products. It is used to thicken drinks, yogurt, cheese, canned food, frozen fruit, pies, jellies, salad dressings, sauces, confectionary and more. May be made from genetically modified plants. No known adverse effects noted in sources, needs more testing. Listed for UK, AU, NZ, EU and USA. Not listed for CAN.
E1451 **Acetylated oxidised starch.** Stabilizing agent,	Made by treating starch with sodium hypochlorite and acetic anhydride. Mostly used in soft gummy candies, but can be used to thicken drinks, yogurt, cheese, canned food, frozen fruit, pies, jellies, salad dressings, sauces, and confectionary May be made from genetically modified plants. No adverse effects listed in sources, needs more testing. Listed for UK and EU. Not listed for AU, NZ, CAN and USA.

Thickening agent, Emulsifier (mixing agent), Binding agent.	
E1452 **Starch Aluminium Octenyl Succinate** Stabilizing agent, Thickening agent.	Aluminum salt from the reaction product of octenylsuccinic anhydride with starch. Mostly used as a thickener for sun creams and other personal care items. Caution with too much intake of manmade aluminum as this may be toxic over time, could be related to senility, memory problems, kidney problems, neurological problems, and also mineral malabsorption. Not much information. Listed for UK.
E1501 **Benzylated hydrocarbons.**	There are three different kinds of Benzylated hydrocarbons. 1. Benzyl alcohol 2. Benzyl acetate 3. Benzyl benzoate All three are made by chemical synthesis for commercial usage. Benzyl alcohol is used as a solvent.

Flavoring agent (sweetener).	Benzyl acetate is a flavoring agent that gives a pear or apple flavor. Benzyl benzoate is another flavoring agent. These three are found in many food products; they are also used in cosmetics and pharmaceuticals. Acceptable daily intake: Up to 5 mg per kg of body weight. No known side effects when used in foods, but skin problems may occur when used in cosmetics, not much information. Not listed for UK, AU, NZ, EU, USA and CAN.
E1502 **Butane-1,3-diol or 1,3-Butanediol.** Solvent (puts chemicals into solution with each other).	$C_4H_{10}O_2$ It is made by chemical synthesis for commercial usage. It is a type of alcohol. It is a viscous liquid, used as a solvent for food flavoring agents. A main use is in tobacco products. Acceptable daily intake is up to 4 mg per kg of body weight. No adverse effects listed in sources, not much information. Not listed for UK, NZ, AU, EU, USA and CAN.
E1503 **Castor Oil.**	C57H104O9 Castor oil is a vegetable oil obtained from the castor bean. It is a liquid that is colorless to very pale yellow with mild odor and taste. Used in foods as a mold inhibitor and as a flavor-carrying agent, can be used as a laxative, but may cause discomfort

Solvent (puts chemicals into solution with each other), Preservative (anti mold and anti fungal), Flavoring agent (carries flavors).	due to cramps and explosive diarrhea etc. Used in chewing gum, cocoa, chocolate products, and candies. Acceptable daily intake is up to 0.7 mg per kg of body weight. No adverse side effects noted in sources with proper usage. Not listed for UK, AU, NZ and EU. Allowed in CAN and USA.
E1504 **Ethyl Acetate** Solvent (puts chemicals into solution with each other), Flavoring agent (carries flavors).	$C_4H_8O_2$ It is a natural component inside many fruits, synthesized for industry mainly by a esterification reaction of ethanol and acetic acid. It is manufactured on a large scale due to low cost and low toxicity. Used in candies, ice cream and cakes. Acceptable daily intake is up to 6 mg per kg of body weight. Ethyl Acetate can be a skin irritant, a nervous system depressant, long-term inhalation of ethyl acetate fumes may cause kidney and liver damage. This condition may cause secondary infections. Not listed for UK, EU, AU, and NZ. Listed for CAN and USA.
E1505	It is commercially made from citric acid, used as a whipping aid,

Triethyl acetate or citrate. Stabilizing agent, Flavoring agent (sour flavor)	thickener, vegetable gum for flavored beverages and sports drinks. It may interfere with medical lab results. Listed for UK, AU, NZ, EU, USA and CAN.
E1510 **Ethanol or Ethyl alcohol, Pure alcohol, Grain alcohol, Drinking alcohol,** Anti-microbial agent, Solvent	CH_3CH_2OH Common drinking alcohol made by fermentation of sugar, afterward if wanted it can be concentrated by distillation. Used in baked goods, alcohol containing candy, sauces, vegetable oil sprays, alcoholic beverages such as whisky, fruit wines, cough syrups and medicines, mouth washes, antiseptics, apple cider, and hairspray etc. Fatal in large dosages, causes cancer in rats and destroys brain cells. It is an addictive substance for some people, if they tend to drink too much it is best to avoid, small amounts on occasion is not that harmful, however alcoholics should avoid. It is safe for proper usage in medicine and foods.

(puts chemicals into solution with each other).	Not listed for UK, AU, NZ and EU. Listed for CAN and USA.
E1516 **Glycerol monoacetate** **or Glycerol monoacetin.** Solvent (puts chemicals into solution with each other), Flavoring agent	$C_5H_{10}O_4$ Glycerol monoacetate is commercially made from acetic acid and glycerol. It is an oily liquid with a bitter taste and fatty odor, used as a solvent to help mix in flavors. It is slightly soluble in water, but very soluble in alcohol. It is used for chocolates, cocoa, and candy. Glycerol is a sugar alcohol, for sensitive people it may cause bloating, laxative effect and diarrhea. It may cause carbohydrate cravings. Not listed for UK, AU, NZ, EU and USA. Listed for CAN.
E1517 **Glycerol diacetate.** Solvent (puts chemicals into solution with each other), Flavoring agent, Anti	$C_7H_{12}O_5$ Glycerol diacetate is commercially made from acetic acid and glycerol. It is an oily liquid with a bitter taste and fatty odor, used as a solvent to mix in flavors. It is soluble in water, but only slightly soluble in alcohol. It is used in medicine cream as an anti fungal agent, also used in butter and cigarette filters. In sensitive people it may cause headaches, nausea,

Fungal agent.	vomiting, dehydration, diarrhea, thirst, dizziness and mental confusion Not listed for UK, AU, NZ, EU and USA. Listed for CAN.
E1518 **Glycerol triacetate or Triacetin or 1,2,3-triacetoxypropane.** Solvent (puts chemicals into solution with each other), Humectant (Water holding agent), Plasticizer (improves fluidity of mixtures).	$C_9H_{14}O_6$ It is the triester of glycerol and acetic acid. It is slightly soluble in water, but very soluble in alcohol. It is an oily liquid with a bitter taste, used as a solvent to mix in flavors. It is used in pharmaceuticals, butter, cosmetics, and cigarette filters etc. Glycerol is a sugar alcohol, for sensitive people it may cause bloating, laxative effect and diarrhea. It may cause carbohydrate cravings. Listed for UK, AU, NZ, EU, USA and CAN.
E1519	$C_6H_5CH_2OH$ Benzyl alcohol is an organic compound that is found naturally in plants and fruits. It is commercially

Benzyl alcohol. Solvent (puts chemicals into solution with each other).	made by the hydrolysis of benzyl chloride using sodium hydroxide. A colorless liquid that is used as a solvent in food products. Benzyl alcohol is used as a bacteriostatic preservative at low concentration in intravenous medications. In healthy individuals it is oxidized rapidly to benzoic acid, conjugated with glycine in the liver, and excreted as hippuric acid. High concentrations can result in toxic effects including respiratory failure, hypotension, convulsions, and paralysis. It is a eye, skin and mucus membrane irritant that may cause diarrhea and vomiting. Newborns, especially if critically ill, may not metabolize benzyl alcohol well enough or at all. Reports in the early 1980s of sixteen neonatal deaths associated with the use of saline flush solutions containing benzyl alcohol preservative led to recommendations to avoid its use for small infants. Used in cosmetics and foods, sensitive adults may have an reaction to low concentrations. Not listed for UK, AU, NZ and EU. Listed for CAN and USA.
E1520	$C_3H_8O_2$ Propylene glycol is commercially made from propylene and carbonate. It is a colorless, nearly odorless, clear

Propylene glycol or 1,2-propanediol or Propane-1,2-diol. Solvent (puts chemicals into solution with each other), Humectant (Water holding agent), Stabilizing agent, Anti-microbial agent (anti fungal, anti bacterial agent), Emulsifier (mixing agent)	viscous liquid with a faintly sweet taste. Used in automobile antifreeze, danger to animals and children, if spilled its sweet taste can encourage drinking. Skin and eye irritant, ingestion in concentrated form can cause kidney pain and failure, blindness, convulsions and death. It is linked to fatal heart attacks when given intravenously. For sensitive people it can cause ill effects at low concentrations (I personally had a kidney attack that came about from toothpaste with Propylene glycol in it. I do have sensitive kidneys) The USA has placed a total recall of any medication containing this additive yet it is still permitted in food. It may be used as a coating on fruit, in margarine, baked goods, poultry, seasonings, alcoholic beverages, flavorings, wine, frostings, frozen dairy products, candy, chocolates, chewing gum, any prepared food and vegetables, nut products, including artificial sweetener bases. It is a carrier liquid for food colors and flavorings. Listed for UK, AU, NZ, EU, USA and CAN.
E1521	$C_{2n}H_{4n+2}O_{n+1}$ Polyethylene glycol is made by the interaction of ethylene oxide with water, ethylene glycol, or ethylene

Polyethylene glycol Or polyethylene oxide (PEO) or polyoxyethylene (POE) or Under trade name Carbowax Solvent (puts chemicals into solution with each other), Humectant (Water holding agent), Emulsifier (mixing agent), Artificial sweetener, Anti foaming agent.	glycol oligomers. Used in chewing gum, food supplements, coating agent for fruits, as a tabletop sweetener and in water-based flavored drinks, including sport drinks, energy drinks, and electrolyte drinks. It is used as a cooling agent in beers, wines and as an emulsifier in orange bitters. Many medical usages including eye drops, laxatives, ointment base, some research suggests it can aid with nerve regeneration. It can be a skin and eye irritant, mildly toxic when ingested, can break down to formaldehyde. It is known to cause renal (kidney) failure in some instances during medical use. Listed for UK, AU, NZ, EU, USA and CAN.
E1524	Hydroxy ethyl cellulose is commercially made from ethanol and

Hydroxy ethyl cellulose. Emulsifier (mixing agent), Stabilizing agent,Thickening agent.	cellulose. Used for food packaging and edible films and coatings. It is widely used in cosmetics, cleaning solutions, and other household products. Acceptable daily intake is up to 25 mg per kg of body weight. It has no known side effects with normal usage as a food additive. In high concentrations, it acts as a laxative. Not listed for UK, AU, NZ, CAN and USA.

Genetically altered foods

In around the mid 1990's there was a rush to genetically alter many kinds of foods. Safeguards to prevent harmful genetic alterations are weak. Of course, genetic changes can be both beneficial for food production and also harmful due to adverse reactions to the final product. In effect, we have an ongoing live experiment on the world's population with genetic engineering of food crops. I expect that there will be many people chronically sick because of this practice.

The Grocery Manufacturers of America estimate that 75 % of all processed foods in the U.S. contain a GM ingredient.

Some estimates there are as 30,000 different products on grocery store shelves are "modified."

Altered genes in foods can cause altered genes in intestinal flora.

To be fair careful genetic engineering can be beneficial, by making disease and pest resistant crops or by adding in vitamins such as vitamin A into rice. There is great potential in medicine to prevent and treat diseases by genetic engineering. The main concern about genetic engineering is that it is profit driven without enough safeguards. That industry can have too much influence on government. There are innumerable possible bad outcomes due to genetic alterations, which may be irreversible.

The most practical concern of today is people made sick by reactions to modified foods. People can be made ill by bad effects that are so slight and slow coming on that they cannot tell why. Many people will end up taking pills and other treatments for illnesses that are not addressing the real cause.

There is practically no risk of jail time for a GMO food producer, there is only profit or loss. You are mostly on your own to protect yourself and your family from GM's allowed in food. Like most anything harmful, most people usually can handle a little and shake it off, but if too much then sickness begins. For a few people traces of something adverse will cause major sickness.

Most developed nations do not consider all GM's safe. Nearly 50 countries, including Australia, Japan, and all of the European Union, restrict or ban the import, production and sale of GMO foods. Food is involved in a large import export market and many nations are not so interested in profits for international companies as they are in safety. This helps moderate the use of GMO foods somewhat. Many GMO foods that could have been put on domestic markets, but has been stopped because of this situation. Just recently in May 2013 GMO wheat from a Oregon USA field has been found in a international wheat shipment, causing an international uproar. GMO producers sometimes study GMO strains using farm fields and it is a concern that they can spread and live on after the tests. Tests with GMO wheat in fields started in 1998 and said to be ended in 2005...

Even though a food may not be GMO, conventional cross breeding can change the nature of foods. Use of cross breeding created hybrids in the 1950's onward greatly increasing food production of single crops in large fields while using fertilizer, herbicides and pesticides This practice has increased the production of commercial foods, but there are serious concerns including food safety, the existence of small farms, *sustainability*, environmental damage and nutrition.

Labeling of fresh fruits and vegetables

You can tell if foods are commercially or organically grown or GMO. Just look at the item itself, or on the pricing on the food stand, for a four or five digit number.

Four digits, it is conventionally grown.
Five digits, starting with the number 8, then genetically modified.
Five digits, starting with the number 9, then organic.

A list of some genetically altered foods (I am dependent on my sources being accurate)

Rapeseed: Before genetic engineering of rapeseed to make Canola (Canadian Oil), rapeseed oil could not be used for consumption due to erucic acid and glucosinolates, which are toxic. Rapeseed is naturally resistant to pests and relativity easy to grow in quantity. Many years ago, industry tried to feed people rapeseed oil, but it was too toxic. Canola oil is a few decades old genetic engineering creation from the rapeseed plant. Recently it has become a popular cheap oil for processed foods and in restaurants. Its human history as a food oil is very short.

Honey: Bees gather nectar to make honey; this can be from genetically modified crops. This honey made from GM nectar is banned from use in Europe. Bees also gather pollen, which is used as food. In recent year's large die offs of honey bees is a warning sign. A possible cause is toxins inside genetically engineered plants. Bees also can die off due to pesticides or natural diseases.

Cotton: Cottonseed oil ranks third in volume behind soybean and corn oil with about 5-6% of the total USA fat and oil supply. Cottonseed is considered a vegetable and it is inside vegetable oil. The plant is resistant to damage by certain pesticides. It can be genetically engineered to control the cotton bollworm. In India after harvest, farmers let livestock graze on the crop remains, with the genetically engineered BT cotton they get sick and die. Cotton has a relatively short history of usage as a food item.

Rice: It can be genetically engineered to contain vitamin A. Other genetic engineering is possible. For example, rice can be made with human genes to be used as medicine on infants with diarrhea.

Soybean: It is genetically engineered to be resistant to herbicides. It makes up about half of the world's edible oil consumption. It is considered a vegetable and can be inside vegetable oil. It is used in many processed food products. Ninety-eight percent of the U.S. soybean crop is used for livestock feed. Rats fed with high amounts of GM soy tend to go sterile by the third generation and their baby mortality is very high. Researchers note that GM soy has a double threat of higher herbicide content (because it is created to be herbicide resistant), along with possible side effects from the genetic engineering.

Tomatoes: Can be GMO altered for longer shelf life, to prevent rot and decay. Rats were fed FlavrSavr (Trademark) GM tomatoes for twenty-eight days. Seven out of twenty had bleeding stomachs and seven out of forty died within two weeks; those tomatoes went off the market due to public outcry. Today no GMO tomatoes are on the market due to public resistance, but research is on going.

Corn: Altered to be resistant to certain pesticides, GM corn often has pesticide built right into the plant's genetics to control insects. Corn is in use to make corn oil and cornstarch and is inside countless processed products. Excessive ingestion of sugar made from corn can lead to diabetes. Corn is in use to feed livestock, to fatten beef or pork before slaughter as feed for dairy cattle. About 1995 onward corn allergies have increased in the human population. About half of the sweet corn planted in the USA (2013-14) is GM. I often have a bad reaction to non-organic corn products. This started for me in around 2004, I had no problems before this time. For example if I eat very much of non-organic cornbread I may be sick for two to three days!

Vegetable oil: It can contain corn oil, soybean oil, canola oil and cotton oil; all of these are GMO. Most North America restaurants use one of these oils individually or together in the form of vegetable oil. Unless these oils are labeled organic they are likely GMO.

Potatoes: There are no GM potatoes on the market due to public resistance and a lack of commercial advantage in prior attempts. There is on going research to create blight resistant potatoes and change its starch make up for ease of commercial processing. Expect more and more GM potatoes for livestock feed and possibly in the human food supply.

Flax: Herbicide-resistant GM flax was introduced in 2001, but was taken off the market because European importers refused to buy it.

Wheat: No GMO wheat on the market today, but research is going on.

Strawberries: Some people think commercially grown strawberries are GMO, but they are not (to date, Nov 2013). However, a concern is the herbicides and pesticides used on crops, which may cause adverse reactions.

Papaya - The first virus resistant papayas were commercially grown in Hawaii in 1999. Today GM papayas make up about three quarters of the total Hawaiian papaya crop. It is said by some sources that without GMO papayas the papaya virus would have destroyed the papaya industry.

Squash: Some zucchini and yellow crookneck squash are also GMO. About 13% of zucchini crops were GMO in USA in 2005 in order to resist viruses. However, the GM virus resistant squash are more vulnerable to insects and bacteria diseases making it less popular for some farmers. There is on going research.

Meat: Meat and dairy often come from animals that have eaten GMO feed. Two main GMO feeds are corn and soybeans. It is better to buy organic and free-range-which is meat not fattened by grain. Naturally grown and grass fed livestock is better for health to eat but has tougher leaner meat.

Peas: GMO peas caused immune responses in mice, suggesting they may create allergic reactions for people. Those GM peas had been made with a gene from kidney beans, which creates a protein that acts as a pesticide. GMO peas are not on the market to date, but there is on going research.

Vegetable Oil - Most vegetable oils and margarines used in restaurants and in processed foods in North America are made from soy, corn, canola, or cottonseed. Unless these oils specifically say "Non-GMO" or "Organic," they are probably genetically modified. Industry says that the final product of these GMO oils have very little to zero of the modified proteins.

Sugarbeet: Sugar beets are main source of sugar and is in many processed products. After deregulation in 2005, a GMO glyphosate-resistant sugar beet became greatly used in the United States. After 2011, about 95% of all USA sugarbeet crops are GMO. Pulp from the refining process is used as animal feed.

Dairy Products: Around 22% of USA cows are injected with GMO altered bovine growth hormone. Livestock, which produce dairy products, are often fed with GMO foods. Most livestock is injected with antibiotics. Growth hormones are used on livestock as well and is passed on to humans. If you eat dairy consider buying organic.

Public resistance to GMO foods has slowed down this industry somewhat. It can be costly and risky in a financial sense for companies to introduce GMO foods. Many people believe it best to buy organic to avoid GMO foods and the most harmful additives and pesticides. However, due to the cost of organic produce many of us cannot buy it or even find it in local stores. Most non-organic foods not given on the list above are not GMO, but still can have pesticide residues and lower in nutrition due to lack organic fertilizer.

As a practical manner, it is important to avoid certain key non-organic products if on a limited food budget. A short list of the most important GMO foods for me to avoid is corn, soybeans, canola and vegetable oil. I also avoid other foods, but usually for other reasons, mostly because of food additives. If you are on tight food budget, it is acceptable to buy non-organic produce and scrub it when you get home. GMO foods, pesticides, herbicides and food additives will change into the future and industry may hide what it is doing to avoid public resistance.

Neurotoxins

A neurotoxin is something that harms the nervous system or the cells in the nervous system. There are many neurotoxins inside of processed foods. Something to consider if you are having neurological health problems such as MS, Parkinson's, Alzheimer's , etc.

Neurotoxins that are food additives

Aspartame	Beef stock
Autolyzed anything	Bouillon
Barley malt	Broth of any kind
Beef base	Beef flavoring
Calcium Caseinate	Chicken broth

Carrageenan	Chicken flavoring
Caseinate	Chicken stock
Chicken base	Disodium anything
Dough conditioner	Flavoring
Malted anything	Seasoning
Milk solids	Smoke flavoring
Monosodium Glutamate	Sodium Caseinate
Natural flavor	Hydrolyzed anything
Nutrasweet	Kombu extract
Pork base	L-cysteine
Pork flavoring	Malt anything
Protein concentrate	Gelatinized anything
Protein extract	Glutamate
Seasoned salt	Gaur gum
Solids of any kind	Spice
Soup base	Stock
Soy extract	Soy protein anything
Soy sauce	Gelatin
Textured protein	Vegetable gum
Textured vegetable protein	Whey anything
Umami	Yeast extract

There are other toxins that are related to neurotoxins, they are called a excitotoxins. Excitotoxins are remarkable in that they cause nerve cells to fire themselves to death. A person may feel a high as their brain nerve cells are excited to death.

Aspartame is a sweetener used in many products. It is a neurotoxin/excitotoxin and when combined with caffeine it has a greater damaging effect. Diet soda is a common example of aspartame combined with caffeine. This soda can cause neurological disease and brain damage, especially when used in excess. Most artificial sweeteners have potential to cause illness, it is best to limit or avoid them.

All the MSG's or hydrolyzed proteins are nurotoxins/excitotoxins. Up to 80% of all processed food products have some kind of MSG (MSG has many different forms, names and variations). It gives foods a savory meaty taste; therefore it is a favorite of consumers and food producers. To avoid most of MSG family don't ingest Glutamate, Glutamic acid, Autolyzed-*anything*, Hydrolyzed-*anything*, *anything*-Protein, *anything*-Flavoring and Carrageenan. Up to 60% of products labeled with *natural flavors* may have some kind of MSG. In avoiding MSG it is best to stay away from processed products especially those with a savory taste. Examples are sauces, chips, gravies and soups etc.

Neurotoxins and excitotoxins are possible direct causes for neurological diseases such as Lou Gehrig's, MS and Parkinson's etc. It often takes up to 80% of nerve cells to be damaged or dead in a given area to have notable symptoms disease. Major damage can occur in childhood and adulthood with no obvious symptoms. Low blood sugar and high temperature during a fever may cause nerve cell damage at a great rate.

An imaginary example is a child sick with fever and low blood sugar due to lack of appetite. Then eats a meal high in neurotoxins (MSG filled canned soup) and this causes a wave of nerve cell damage. However no sign of nerve cell damage yet, but as the years go by and further damage adds up until he or she develops nervous system disease. This depends on the individual as certain people are more sensitive than others.

Another imaginary example is a runner in their forties who pushes too hard in a long hot race, (high body temperature and low blood sugar) thereby killing off the last bit of extra nerve cells before the onset of illness. Do not give infants aspirin when sick because it can cause low blood sugar, therefore nerve cell damage.

If sick with nerve degeneration disease or have a family history of nervous system disease, it is extra important to avoid neurotoxins and excitotoxins in foods, drinks and environment. Avoid the MSG family of additives, artificial sweeteners and chemicals in general. If feeling the onset of nervous system disease avoid being low in blood sugar, which increases nerve cell damage, or being over heated while physically stressed. First thing in the morning, consider eating a healthy grain, such as oatmeal, organic corn or brown rice. To give a steady supply of glucose for the brain's energy needs. It is most important to avoid heat stroke conditions and extreme exercise. Be sure to get enough magnesium in the diet, consider taking a magnesium supplement, which protects the nervous system. Avoid vaccines and toxic metals such as aluminum, lead and mercury, remove mercury containing dental fillings, and limit eating sugar, the MSG family of additives and artificial sweeteners. Limit high glycemic foods, processed foods, pesticide laden non-organic foods and toxic personal care products such as unclean toothpaste, lotions, cosmetics and antiperspirants. Make sure the illness is not related to unknown viruses, bacteria or parasites, see chapter twenty in "The King's Table" for anti pathogen treatments. For more information find "Excitotoxins-The Taste that Kills" by Russell Blaylock, M.D.

Some "natural" products can be dangerously neurotoxic as well. An example is tea tree oil, which is a strong neurotoxin. One must be careful in usage of strong natural remedies, especially if something natural is concentrated. It is best to use strong remedies carefully and cycle off and on, as needed. One may use mild herbal remedies long term (if needed) while carefully monitoring their effect on the body watching for bad side effects. Many people into being healthy overdo natural remedies and treatments. Sometimes these mistakes are damaging and irreversible, do your homework and research proper usage of any natural substance. I am leery of pharmaceuticals, especially those new on the market, for instance less than ten years. The wise person will do their own research about side effects for any medicine or remedy. The best medicine is good clean food and drink with positive lifestyle.

With most anything harmful some people are more sensitive. If you have signs of nervous system disease it is extra important to clean up the diet. Symptoms are the inability to think normally or move the body properly. See a Naturopath or Ecological doctor and do more research. Remember there is opposing information about health subjects on the internet, news, science research and universities, so crosscheck all information.

Most of us know that food additives, herbs, supplements and pharmaceuticals can cause adverse reactions. What is not well known is that other ingredients rather than the prime active ingredient can cause adverse reactions. These fillers, binders or other active ingredients that may vary from one batch or brand of pills to the next. Here is a list of some common ones.

Other ingredients inside of pharmaceuticals or pills (fillers, binders, etc)

Propylene Glycol (anti freeze)	Calcium phosphate
Sucrose	Sodium Starch Glycolate
Povidone	Pregelatinized Starch
Hydroxy Propyl Methycellulose	Stearic Acid
Calcium Stearate	
Microcrystalline	Ethylcellulose
Cellulose	Lactose (milk sugar)
Silicon Dioxide	Starch
BHT	Polysorbate 80

BHA	Peanut Oil
Cellulose	Hydroxy Propyl Cellulose
Tartrazine	Microcrystalline
Red Dye 33 and 40	Hydrogenated Cottonseed Oil
Fractionated Coconut Oil	Ethyl Cellulose
Sodium Benzoate	Fractionated Cornstarch

Anything that you ingest can be toxic for you. It is difficult in modern life to live and consume without worry. Just now, as I am writing these lines, I am having a bad reaction from a natural food that I bought from a health food store. I am having a feeling of sickness for a full day. I suspect a type of dried fruit from the natural food bins. What I bought is labeled organic, but I am suspicious there may be food additives. It is difficult to figure out the exact cause because I am eating several different dried fruits and raw nuts. I wonder am I having an allergic reaction to something natural or it's because of an unnatural food additive? Out of necessity I do not blindly trust foods, even those labeled organic.

In modern life we must be cautious of anything ingested, especially long term. Do not blindly use cosmetics, lotions, soaps and anything smelly. They may create a toxic build up and destroy health. Most any kind of illness can be caused by toxins, including diseases with mysterious causes. Possibilities are liver failure, gall bladder failure, kidney failure, organ failure of any kind and cancer.

Fetuses inside the womb, infants and small children are more sensitive to toxins. In modern life people use many types of personal care products. Most of these are made overseas by the lowest bidder and imported, almost all made with chemicals. Check the labels and find many chemical names, each is a potential toxin that may cause cancer, nervous system damage, hormonal changes and more.

For an imaginary example, take the mother who uses her favorite lotion for years. Now her skin must have it to be moist, it is an addictive relationship. Then she becomes pregnant and toxins from the lotion are around the fetus during it's development. If there are *gender bender* hormonal toxins the baby may have opposing gender identity influences long before it is born. After birth the mother may use her favorite lotion on the baby's skin where it is absorbed. Babies being physically immature are unable to remove toxins as well as adults.

Most any kind of damage is possible from chemicals inside personal care products, neurotoxin damage, hormonal effects, adverse physical and mental defects, damage to sex organs and cancer. Many people use air fresheners, soaps, cosmetics and lotions with very little thought...

Look inside the average home and you will see a witches brew of chemicals, inside products and building materials. Chemicals when absorbed through skin and breathed in have quicker access inside of the body than toxins in foods that must go past the liver, which is a detoxification organ. The effect is stronger for those people who are sensitive.

Use a slightly toxic product months, years, to decades (maybe a addictive relationship) it can work to destroy health. The same consideration with any kind of toxin emitting from the home such as mold spores or chemical fumes off glue filled building products. Toxic affects may not be sudden, but come on slow and destroy health.

A good procedure is to look at a product's label, then look up its ingredients. If there is an indication of toxic effect then reflect how often you use the product and if worth the risk. You may be able to find better replacements in cosmetics, lotions, perfumes and soaps. Here is a list of potential toxins in personal care products. How toxic each can be depends on individual genetics and how often used. Some may not be toxic except for individuals who have an allergic reaction.

Possible toxins that may be in personal care products.

Acesulfame:		Toxin-carcinogen
Acid Blue 9:	color;	Toxin-allergen
Acid Orange:	color;	Toxin-allergen
Acid Yellow 6:	color;	Toxin-allergen
Acid Yellow 10:	color;	Toxin-allergen
Acid Yellow 17:	color;	Toxin-allergen
Acid Yellow 23:	color;	Toxin-allergen
Acrylamide:		Toxin-carcinogen
Acrylate polymer:		Toxin
Alpha-hydroxy acid:		Penetration enhancer
Alpha-hydroxycaprylic acid:		Penetration enhancer
Alpha-hydroxyethanoic acid:		Penetration enhancer
Alpha-hydroxyoctanoic acid:		Penetration enhancer
Armica:	toners;	Toxin-allergen
Arnica:	toners;	Toxin-allergen
Ammonium thioglycolate:	hair waving solution;	Toxin-allergen
Amorphous silicates:		Potential toxin
Aryl sulfonamide:	nail varnish;	Toxin-allergen
Aspartame:		Toxin-carcinogen
Auramine:		Toxin-carcinogen
Avobenzone:		Hormone disrupter
Benzalkonium chloride:		preservative; Toxin-allergen
Benzophenene-3, (BP3):		sunscreens; Toxin-allergen
Benzylparaben:		Hormone disrupter
Benzyl salicylate:	sunscreens;	Toxin-allergen

Benzyl alcohol:	face creams;	Toxin-allergen
Beta-hydroxybutanoic acid:	Penetration enhancer	
Bisabolol:	Penetration enhancer	
Bisphenol-A (BPA):	Toxin-carcinogen	
Blue 2:	coal tar dye;	Toxin-carcinogen
Butadiene:	Toxin-carcinogen	
Butane:	Potential toxin	
Butylbenzyl phthalate:	Toxin-carcinogen	
Butylated hydroxyanisole (BHA):		
	Toxin-carcinogen	
Butylmethoxydibenzoylmethane (BMDM):		
	Hormone disrupter	
Butylparaben:	Hormone disrupter	
Brononitrodioxane:	Potential toxin	
Bronopol:	Potential toxin	
Castor oil:	lipsticks;	Toxin-allergen
Cetyl alcohal:	face creams;	Toxin-allergen
Chromium trioxide:	Toxin-carcinogen	
Cinnamic salicylate:	deodorants;	Toxin-allergen
Citric acid:	Penetration enhancer	
Coal tar dye:	Potential toxin	
Cobalt chloride:	Toxin-carcinogen	
Cocamidopropyl betaine:	Potential toxin	
Colophony:	lipsticks;	Toxin-allergen
Condenstates:	Potential toxin	
Coumarin:	toners;	Toxin-allergen
Cyclamates:	Toxin-carcinogen	
D&-C:	coal tar dye;	Toxin-carcinogen
Diaminophenol:	Toxin-carcinogen	
Diazolidinyl urea:	preservative;	Toxin-allergen
Dibutyl phthalate (DBP):	Hormone disrupter	
Diethyl phthalate (DEP):	Hormone disrupter	
Diethanolamine (DEA):		

Toxin-carcinogen/penetration enhancer	
DEA and fatty acid condensates:	
	Potential toxin
DEA cocamide condensate:	Toxin-carcinogen
DEA oleamide condensate:	Toxin-carcinogen
DEA sodium lauryl sulfate:	Toxin-carcinogen
Diethylhexyl phthalate (DEHP):	Toxin-carcinogen
Dimethyl phthalate (DMP):	Hormone disrupter
Dioctyl adipate:	Toxin-carcinogen
Dioctyl phthalate (DEHP):	Hormone disrupter
Disodium ethylenediamine tetra-acetic acid (EDTA):	
	Hormone disrupter/penetration enhancer
Disperse yellow 3:	Toxin-carcinogen
DMDM hydatoin: preservative;	Toxin-allergen
Esthylenediamine: preservative;	Toxin-allergen
Ethylenediamine tetra-acetic acid (EDTA):	
	Hormone disrupter/penetration enhancer
Ethyl methacrylate: preservative;	Toxin-allergen
Ethylparaben:	Hormone disrupter
FD&C: coal tar dye;	Toxin-carcinogen
FD&C Blue 2: color;	Toxin-allergen
FD&C Red 2: color;	Toxin-allergen
FD&C Yellow 6: color;	Toxin-allergen
Formaldehyde:	Toxin-carcinogen
Fragrances or perfumes:	Toxins-allergens
Glutaral:	Toxin-carcinogen
Glyceryl laurate:	Penetration enhancer
Glyceryl thioglycolate:	hair waving solution;
	Toxin-allergen
Glycolic acid:	Penetration enhancer
Glycolic acid and ammonium glycolate:	
	Penetration enhancer

Glyoxal:		Potential toxin
Green 3:	coal tar dye;	Toxin-carcinogen
Green 5:	coal tar dye;	Toxin-carcinogen
Henna:	color;	Toxin-allergen
Homosalate (HMS):		Hormone disrupter
Hulsam of peru:	deodorant;	Toxin-allergen
Hydroquinone:		Toxin-carcinogen
Hydroxycaprylic acid:		Penetration enhancer
Imidazolidinyl urea:		preservative; Toxin-allergen
Lactic acid:		Penetration enhancer
Jasmine:	deodorant;	Toxin-allergen
L-alpha-hydroxy acid:		Penetration enhancer
Lanolin:		Toxin-allergen
Laureth - alchohal ethoxylate:		Potential toxin
Lead:		Toxin-carcinogen
Limonene:		Toxin-carcinogen
Malic acid:		Penetration enhancer
Methacrylate polymer:		Potential toxin
Metheneamine:		Toxin-carcinogen
Methyl anisate:	deodorant;	Toxin-allergen
4-Methyl-benzylidine camphor (4-MBC):		Hormone disrupter
Methyl methacrylate:		artificial nails; Toxin-allergen
Methylparaben:		Hormone disrupter
Methylene chloride:		Toxin-carcinogen
Methyldibromoglutaronitrile:		preservative; Toxin-allergen
Mineral oils:		Toxin-carcinogen
Mixed fruit acid:		Penetration enhancer
Monoethanolamine:		Penetration enhancer
Morpholine:		Potential toxin

Nitrofurazone:	Toxin-carcinogen
Nonoxynols - phenol ethoxylates:	Potential toxin
Nonylphenol (NP):	Hormone disrupter
Oak moss: toners;	Toxin-allergen
Octinoxatc:	Hormone disrupter
Octoxynols - phenol ethoxylates:	Potential toxin
Octyl-dimethyl-paba (OD-PABA):	
	Hormone disrupter
Octyl-methoxycinnamate (OMC):	
	Hormone disrupter
Oleth - alchohal ethoxylate:	Potential toxin
Orange 17:	Toxin-carcinogen
Oxybenzone: sunscreens;	Toxin-allergen
Padimate-O:	Potential toxin
Palmitic acid:	Penetration enhancer
Para-aminobenzoic acid (PABA):	sunscreens;
	Toxin-allergen
Parabens: (Inside of many personal care products, often not labeled);	
	Toxin-allergen
Petroleum:	Potential toxin
p-Phenylenedimine (ppd):	hair dye;
	Toxin-allergen
Phenol formaldehyde resin:	nail base coat;
	Toxin-allergen
Phenylenediamines:	Toxin-carcinogen
Pigments: cosmetics-colorings;	Toxin-allergen
Polyacrylamide:	Potential toxin
Poly alpha-hydroxy acid:	Penetration enhancer
Polyoxyethylene:	Potential toxin
Polyoxymethylene urea:	Potential toxin
Polysorbates - alcohol exthxylates:	Potential toxin
Polyethylene glycol (PEG) - alcohol ethxylates:	

		Potential toxin
Propyl gallate:	lipsticks;	Toxin-allergen
Propylparaben:		Hormone disrupter
Propylene glycol:	antifreeze;	Toxin-allergen
Pyrocatechol:		Toxin-carcinogen
p-toluenediamine:	hair dye;	Toxin-allergen
Quaternium-15:	preservative;	Toxin-allergen
Quanterniums:		Potential toxin
Red 3,4,8,9,17,19,33, 40:		coal tar dye; Toxin-carcinogen
Red 22, 2G:	color;	Toxin-allergen
Resorcinol:	color;	Toxin-allergen
Saccharin (Sweet N low)@:		Toxin-carcinogen
Salicylic acid:		Penetration enhancer
Sarcosine:		Potential toxin
Silica (crystalline):		Toxin-carcinogen
Sodium hydroxymethylglycinate:		Potential toxin
Sodium lauryl sarcosinate:		Penetration enhancer
Sodium lauryl sulfate:		Penetration enhancer
Solvents:		Toxins-allergens
Sugar cane extract:		Penetration enhancer
Surfactants (These lower interaction resistance between two substances):		Toxins-allergens
Stearic acid:	face creams;	Toxins-allergens
Talc (powder):		Toxin-carcinogen
Thimerosal:	preservative;	Toxin-allergen
Thioglycolate:	depilatories;	Toxin-allergen
Titanium dioxide (powder):		Toxin-carcinogen
Trethocanic acid:		Penetration enhancer
Tri-alpha-hydroxy acid:		Penetration enhancer
Triclocarban:		Hormone disrupter
Triclosan:		Hormone disrupter

Triethanolamine (TEA):		
	Potential toxin/penetration enhancer	
2,5-Toluene diamine:	color;	Toxin-allergen
3,4-Toluene diamine:	color;	Toxin-allergen
Triclosan:	mascaras;	Toxin-allergen
Triple fruit acid:	Penetration enhancer	
Tropic acid:	Penetration enhancer	
Yellow 6:	coal tar dye;	Toxin-carcinogen

List of references

"Food Additives: A Shoppers Guide to What's Safe & What's Not!" by Christine Hoza Farlow. D.C.

http://www.disabled-world.com

http://www.gmo-compass.org

http://www.food.gov.uk/safereating/additivesbranch/enumberlist

http://home.iprimus.com.au/foo7/additiveban.html

http://www.accessdata.fda.gov/scripts/fcn/fcnNavigation.cfm?filter=ethyl+cellulose&sortColumn=&rpt=eafusListing

http://www.fedupwithfoodadditives.info/factsheets/Factcoloursworld.htm#USA

http://www.hc-sc.gc.ca/fn-an/securit/addit/diction/dict_food-alim_add-eng.php#c

http://home.iprimus.com.au/foo7/additiveban.html

http://www.food.gov.uk/

http://www.foodreactions.org/allergy/additives/900.html

http://www.inmotionfitness.com.au/wp-content/uploads/2011/03/Food-Additives-List-Complete.pdf

http://www.mbm.net.au/health/guide.htm

http://www.fooddirive.com/additive/potassium-ferrocyanide

http://www.naturalnews.com

http://www.wikipedia.org/

http://www.doclocke.com

http://www.wnho.net/excitotoxins death by profit margin.pdf

truthinlabeling.org

If you wish, cut these out to put in purses or wallets.

Four digits, it is conventionally grown.
Five digits, starting with the number 8, then genetically modified.
Five digits, starting with the number 9, then organic.

Four digits, it is conventionally grown.
Five digits, starting with the number 8, then genetically modified.
Five digits, starting with the number 9, then organic.

Four digits, it is conventionally grown.
Five digits, starting with the number 8, then genetically modified.
Five digits, starting with the number 9, then organic.

www.ingramcontent.com/pod-product-compliance
Lightning Source LLC
Chambersburg PA
CBHW050107280326
41933CB00010B/1005